GLORIA JEAN SHOVER RN, BSN, AHI

Student Workbook and Resource Guide for

Nursing Basics for Clinical Practice

Connections to Nursing Practice

AUDREY BERMAN PhD, RN, AOCN
SHIRLEE J. SNYDER EdD, RN
DEBRA S. MCKINNEY MSN, MBA/HCM, RN

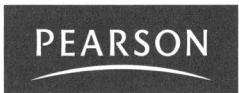

Boston Columbus Indianapolis New York San Francisco Upper Saddle River
Amsterdam Cape Town Dubai London Madrid Milan Munich Paris Montreal Toronto
Delhi Mexico City Sao Paulo Sydney Hong Kong Seoul Singapore Taipei Tokyo

Notice: Care has been taken to confirm the accuracy of information presented in this textbook. The authors, editors, and publisher, however, cannot accept responsibility for errors or omissions or for consequences from application of the information in this textbook and make no warranty, expressed or implied, with respect to its contents.

The authors and publisher have exerted every effort to ensure that drug selections and dosages set forth in this textbook are in accord with current recommendations and practices at the time of publication. However, in view of ongoing research, changes in government regulations, and the constant flow of information relating to drug therapy and drug reactions, the reader is urged to check the package inserts of all drugs for any change in indications of dosage and for added warnings and precautions. This is particularly important when the recommended agent is a new and/or infrequently employed drug.

Publisher: Julie Levin Alexander
Publisher's Assistant: Regina Bruno
Editor-in-Chief: Maura Connor
Acquisitions Editor: Kelly Trakalo
Assistant Editor: Lauren Sweeney
Director of Marketing: David Gesell
Marketing Specialist: Michael Sirinides
Managing Editor for Production: Patrick Walsh
Production Liaison: Yagnesh Jani
Production Editor: Heather Willison, S4Carlisle Publishing Services
Manufacturing Manager: Ilene Sanford
Art Director: Maria Guglielmo-Walsh
Cover Designer: Wanda Espana/Wee Design Group
Composition: S4Carlisle Publishing Services
Cover Printer: Lehigh Phoenix Color/Hagerstown
Printer/Binder: Edwards Brothers

Copyright © 2011 Pearson Education, Inc., Upper Saddle River, New Jersey, 07458.
Pearson Prentice Hall. All rights reserved. Printed in the United States of America. This publication is protected by Copyright and permission should be obtained from the publisher prior to any prohibited reproduction, storage in a retrieval system, or transmission in any form or by any means, electronic, mechanical, photocopying, recording, or likewise. For information regarding permission(s), write to: Rights and Permissions Department.

Pearson® is a registered trademark of Pearson plc

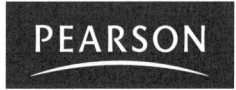

www.pearsonhighered.com

10 9 8 7 6 5 4 3 2 1
ISBN 13: 978-0-13-603550-3
ISBN 10:   0-13-603550-7

Contents

		Preface	v
Chapter	1	Principles of Nursing and Evidence-Based Practice	1
Chapter	2	Legal and Ethical Aspects of Nursing	5
Chapter	3	Health Care Delivery Systems	10
Chapter	4	Culture and Heritage	15
Chapter	5	Health Beliefs and Practices	20
Chapter	6	Critical Thinking and Clinical Reasoning	25
Chapter	7	The Nursing Process	29
Chapter	8	Informatics, Documentation, and Reporting	34
Chapter	9	Promoting Health throughout the Lifespan	39
Chapter	10	Promoting Health in Elders	44
Chapter	11	Promoting Health in the Family	49
Chapter	12	Caring	53
Chapter	13	Communication	57
Chapter	14	Teaching	62
Chapter	15	Leading, Managing, and Delegating	67
Chapter	16	Vital Signs	71
Chapter	17	Health Assessment	76
Chapter	18	Pain Management	81
Chapter	19	Asepsis	87
Chapter	20	Diagnostic Testing	92
Chapter	21	Safety	97
Chapter	22	Hygiene	102
Chapter	23	Medications	107
Chapter	24	Skin Integrity and Wound Care	112

Chapter	25	Perioperative Nursing	118
Chapter	26	Sensory Perception	124
Chapter	27	Self-Concept	128
Chapter	28	Sexuality	132
Chapter	29	Spirituality	137
Chapter	30	Coping with Stress, Loss, and Death	142
Chapter	31	Activity, Exercise, and Sleep	148
Chapter	32	Nutrition	154
Chapter	33	Urinary Elimination	160
Chapter	34	Fecal Elimination	165
Chapter	35	Oxygenation and Circulation	170
Chapter	36	Fluid, Electrolyte, and Acid–Base Balance	176
		Answer Key	181

Preface

Students entering the field of nursing have a tremendous amount to learn in a very short time. This concise student workbook and resource guide has been developed to help you learn and apply key concepts and procedures, and master critical-thinking skills based on *Nursing Basics for Clinical Practice*.

At the beginning of each chapter you will find an Explore MyNursingKit box. Just as in the main textbook this box identifies some specific resources available at www.mynursingkit.com for the chapter. In addition, each chapter includes a variety of questions and activities to help you comprehend difficult concepts and reinforce basic knowledge gained from textbook reading assignments. Highlights of this workbook include:

- Chapters that correlate directly to *Nursing Basics for Clinical Practice* to allow you to easily locate information related to each question.
- Thorough assessment of essential information in the chapter through generous use of matching, short-answer, and multiple-choice questions.
- Matching exercises that contain key terms and definitions from each chapter.
- Multiple choice questions that provide additional review on key topics.
- Thorough assessment of essential information in the text is provided through the Key Topic Review activities.
- Case studies that provide in-depth scenarios to sharpen critical-thinking skills.
- Answers that are included in an appendix to provide immediate reinforcement and allow you to check the accuracy of your work.

It is our hope that this workbook contributes to your success in beginning the study of the exciting and challenging subject of nursing.

CHAPTER 1

PRINCIPLES OF NURSING AND EVIDENCE-BASED PRACTICE

KEY TERM REVIEW

Match each term with its appropriate definition.

1. _____ Client
2. _____ Client advocate
3. _____ Counseling
4. _____ Diagnosis-related groups
5. _____ Environment
6. _____ Evidence-based practice
7. _____ Health
8. _____ Leader
9. _____ Nursing
10. _____ Profession
11. _____ Theory

a. Degree of wellness or well-being that the client experiences

b. Establish pretreatment diagnosis billing categories

c. Process of helping a client to recognize and cope with stressful psychologic or social problems; to promote personal growth

d. Influences others to work together to accomplish a specific goal

e. An occupation that requires extensive education

f. Recipient of nursing care

g. A system of ideas that is proposed to explain given phenomenon

h. Nursing role of pleading the cause of a client

i. Attributes, characteristics, and actions of the nurse providing care on behalf of, or in conjunction with, the client

j. The internal and external surroundings that affect the client

k. The use of substantiation for making clinical decisions

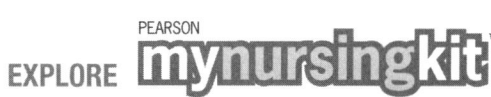

EXPLORE

www.mynursingkit.com

MyNursingKit is your one stop for online chapter review materials and resources. Prepare for success with additional NCLEX®-style practice questions, interactive assignments and activities, web links, animations and videos, and more! Register your access code from the front of your textbook at www.mynursingkit.com

Look for these resources:
- NCLEX® Review
- Case Studies
- Videos and Animations

KEY TOPIC REVIEW

12. List three nursing organizations.

13. List three of the nursing theorists.

14. List areas where a profession is distinguished from other kinds of occupations.

15. List Benner's model describing the five levels of proficiency in nursing.

16. List four of the eight themes that are common to many definitions of nursing.

17. The Henry Street Settlement provided trained nursing services to the poor. Who were the founding nurses?

18. List the four areas that the nurse's practice is involved in.

19. What are the three things that nurses do to help prevent illness?

20. In the United States today, what are the five means of entry into registered nursing?

21. List three areas where hospice nurses work.

22. List examples of tort law that affect nursing.

CASE STUDY

23. A nursing student has just completed four years of school and has received her BSN. She now has to decide what area of nursing she wants to go into. She rotated through all areas but was never comfortable in any of them. Although she enjoys taking care of the patients, she likes to work on computers and make sure all the paperwork is filed correctly. She also enjoys sharing her knowledge and trying to discover why things happen. She plans on taking some time off to look into jobs that are available in her area and to consider how best to spend her time to advance her career.

    1. What medical area will best utilize nursing skills and interest in computers?

    2. What opportunities do nurses have other than direct client care?

    3. Why is it important for nurses to have computer skills?

    4. What benefit would she have if she went back to school?

REVIEW QUESTIONS

24. Who was the nurse known as the "Lady with the Lamp" who helped to reform hospitals?

    a. Clara Barton

    b. Linda Richards

    c. Florence Nightingale

    d. Mary Mahoney

25. Who was the first African American nurse?

    a. Lillian Wald

    b. Mary Mahoney

    c. Linda Richards

    d. Mary Brewster

26. The founder of Planned Parenthood was actually imprisoned for opening the first birth control information clinic. Who was she?

    a. Mary Brewster

    b. Margaret Sanger

    c. Mary Breckinridge

    d. Mary Carnegie

27. Who wrote the theory for redefining nursing as a caring–healing model?

    a. Florence Nightingale

    b. Betty Neuman

    c. Jean Watson

    d. Madeleine Leininger

28. Research for nurses is needed to:

    a. advance the profession.

    b. increase the cost of caring for clients.

    c. provide for job security.

    d. influence students to become nurses.

29. Nursing is best defined as which of the following?

    a. Handmaidens of the physician

    b. Women who wear white

    c. Someone who assists the client in the activities that contribute to health, recovery, or death

    d. Overpaid and undereducated

30. In earlier cultures those that provided care developed special roles that were incorporated into other positions such as which of the following?

    a. Barbers

    b. Priests, witches, and shamans

    c. Butchers

    d. Farmers

31. Houses of care and healing (the first hospitals) were set up in the Roman Empire by which of the following?

    a. Deaconesses

    b. Pope

    c. King

    d. Peasants

32. In protecting the public, each state sets up legal acts to regulate the practice of nursing so all nurses no matter where they work will provide similar standards of care. What are these legal acts called?

    a. Nursing process

    b. Standards of practice

    c. Nurse practice acts

    d. State laws of nursing

33. Who organized nursing services during the Civil War and helped to establish the American Red Cross?

    a. Mary Mahoney

    b. Florence Nightingale

    c. Linda Richards

    d. Clara Barton

34. Who participated in the movement for women's rights and for legislation for nurses to control their own profession?

    a. Lavinia Dock

    b. Mary Brewster

    c. Florence Nightingale

    d. Linda Richards

35. Consumers are now more informed about their health concerns, especially those with chronic health conditions or life-threatening disease. Which of the following is the most common source of information?

    a. Ask a nurse

    b. Internet

    c. Family physician

    d. Health department

36. Schools of nursing traditionally taught students the knowledge and skills to work in a hospital. Now, with new scientific and technical knowledge, curricula have been revised to:

    a. teach more for extended care.

    b. teach for the needs of the community.

    c. meet the needs of nurses in changing environments.

    d. teach whatever the students can absorb.

37. All nursing programs, whether they train practical nursing or registered nursing students, require the approval from which of the following?

    a. Local hospitals

    b. American Medical Association

    c. American Nursing Association

    d. State board of nursing

CHAPTER 2

LEGAL AND ETHICAL ASPECTS OF NURSING

KEY TERM REVIEW

Match each term with its appropriate definition.

1. _____ Advocate
2. _____ Assault
3. _____ Autonomy
4. _____ Battery
5. _____ Beliefs
6. _____ Beneficence
7. _____ Breach of duty
8. _____ Causation
9. _____ Code of ethics
10. _____ Contract
11. _____ Credentialing
12. _____ Defamation
13. _____ Delegation
14. _____ False imprisonment
15. _____ Gross negligence
16. _____ Health care proxy
17. _____ Informed consent
18. _____ Invasion of privacy
19. _____ Liability

a. The process of determining and maintaining competence in the nursing practice

b. The skills and learning commonly possessed by members of a profession to protect the consumer

c. Involves extreme lack of knowledge, skill, or decision making that the person clearly should have known would put others at risk for harm

d. Misconduct or practice that is below the standard expected of an ordinary, reasonable, and prudent person

e. A "professional negligence" that occurred while the person was performing as a professional

f. A standard of care that is expected in the specific situation that the nurse failed to observe

g. An attempt or threat to touch another person unjustifiably

h. The willful touching of a person

i. the "unjustifiable detention of a person without legal warrant to confine the person

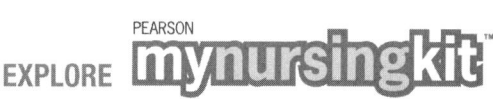

EXPLORE mynursingkit

www.mynursingkit.com

MyNursingKit is your one stop for online chapter review materials and resources. Prepare for success with additional NCLEX®-style practice questions, interactive assignments and activities, web links, animations and videos, and more! Register your access code from the front of your textbook at www.mynursingkit.com

Look for these resources:
- NCLEX® Review
- Case Studies
- Videos and Animations

20. _____ Libel
21. _____ Malpractice
22. _____ Negligence
23. _____ Nonmaleficence
24. _____ Standards of care

j. A direct wrong of a personal nature that injures the feelings of a person and does not take into account the effect of revealed information on the reputation of the person in the community

k. Communication that is false

l. Defamation by means of print, writing, or pictures

m. An agreement, written or oral, between two or more competent persons

n. Nurses' legal responsibility for their obligations and actions and to make financial restitution for wrongful acts

o. An agency record of an accident or unusual occurrence

p. The transfer of responsibility for the performance of an activity from one person to another while retaining accountability for the outcome

q. Also called a durable power of attorney for health care

r. Interpretations or conclusions that people accept as true

s. Refers to the right to make one's own decisions

t. The duty to "do no harm"

u. Means "doing good"

v. Refers to telling the truth

w. A formal statement of a group's ideals and values

x. One who expresses and defends the cause of another

KEY TOPIC REVIEW

25. List three important skills for health professionals.

26. List two ways that nurses would be impaired.

27. Standards of care are used to evaluate the quality of care nurses provide and are legal guidelines for nursing practice. List three internal standards.

28. List the two main types of laws.

29. List the tort laws that affect nurses.

30. What are three areas of unethical conduct?

31. List the three major elements for a client to make an informed decision.

32. List the primary sources of laws in the United States.

33. List the five steps involved in a lawsuit.

34. List three things that credentialing includes.

35. List specialty areas in which nurses receive certification for validating that they have met the minimum standards of nursing.

36. List four internal standards of care for nurses.

37. List the five elements that must be present for a case of nursing malpractice to be proven.

38. List nursing situations in which negligent actions are most likely to occur causing a malpractice suit.

CASE STUDY

39. A client was admitted to the cardiac unit from the emergency department with chest pain. The client was given medications before coming to the unit. The paperwork was held up and the admitting nurse dispensed medication to the client before checking the chart. The client suffered adverse side effects and had to stay in the hospital for an extra week.

    1. What legal action can the client take?
    2. Who is ultimately responsible for financial damages?
    3. What can the hospital do to prevent these errors in the future?
    4. Will the nurse lose her license because of the medication error?

REVIEW QUESTIONS

40. A nurse has been subpoenaed to testify. Before she gives any statements or answers any questions, she should first:

    a. talk to other nurses and see what is expected of her.
    b. talk to her supervisor about her rights when testifying.
    c. talk to her mother about what she should do.
    d. speak with the facility's attorney.

41. A nurse is assigned a client but for unknown reasons has refused to care for "that" patient. This is considered which of the following?

    a. Unethical conduct
    b. Fraud
    c. Breach of confidentiality
    d. Ethical conduct

42. A client admitted to the hospital brought in a large amount of cash and several pieces of expensive jewelry. She decided not to inform the nurse and signed a waiver. When she was being discharged, she noticed some of the cash was missing along with a ring. She notified the nurse to file a complaint. Who is responsible for the loss?

    a. The hospital
    b. The client's personal insurance
    c. The nurse who admitted the client
    d. The client

43. A nurse caring for a client enters into a contract that is which of the following?

    a. Implied consent
    b. Expressed consent
    c. Informed consent
    d. Expected

44. Which of the following is true about the nurse practice acts?

    a. They provide standardized care.
    b. They do not protect the client from harm.
    c. They allow the nurse to write orders independently.
    d. They place responsibility for care on the physician.

45. The doctrine "respondeat superior" means that:

    a. nurses are absolved from criminal acts.
    b. the employer assumes responsibility for nurses' actions.
    c. liability is removed from the nurse.
    d. the nurse is superior over other caregivers.

46. A nurse is encouraged to carry liability insurance because:

    a. nurses can be sued or countersued.
    b. nurses can provide diagnoses for friends.
    c. the insurance can provide job security.
    d. insurance can provide a tax write-off.

47. What does HIPAA stand for?

    a. Health Insurers Probable Accidental Article
    b. Health Inmates Passing Alcoholics Anonymous
    c. Health Insurance Portability and Accountability Act
    d. Health Insurance Providing Anonymity Act

48. Nurses should always be vigilant and observant and need to report any practices that endanger the health and safety of clients. The reporting of these events is referred to as which of the following?

    a. Tattling
    b. Squealing
    c. Testifying
    d. Whistle-blowing

49. Laws that are designed to protect health care providers who offer assistance to a person outside the workplace during a trauma are called which of the following?

    a. Good neighbor acts

    b. Good Samaritan acts

    c. Nurse practice acts

    d. Standards of care

50. A client's medical record is a legal document and can be used in a court case. The usual cause for damages awarded is due to which of the following?

    a. Incompetent care

    b. Negligence

    c. Lack of insurance

    d. Poor documentation

51. Euthanasia is also known as which of the following?

    a. Involuntary death

    b. Mercy killing

    c. Accidental death

    d. A criminal act

52. Which state department oversees the state board of nursing?

    a. ANA

    b. NLN

    c. Department of health

    d. NCSB

CHAPTER 3

HEALTH CARE DELIVERY SYSTEMS

KEY TERM REVIEW

Match each term with its appropriate definition.

1. _____ Case managers
2. _____ Coinsurance
3. _____ Critical pathway
4. _____ Differentiated practice
5. _____ Health care system
6. _____ Health maintenance organization (HMO)
7. _____ Managed care
8. _____ Medicaid
9. _____ Medicare
10. _____ Patient-focused care
11. _____ Preferred provider organization (PPO)
12. _____ Prospective payment system
13. _____ Shared governance model
14. _____ State Children's Health Insurance Program
15. _____ Team nursing

a. The totality of services offered by all health disciplines

b. Function to ensure that clients receive appropriate care; may include a nurse, social worker, occupational therapist, physical therapist, or any other member of the health care team

c. An interdisciplinary plan or tool that specifies interdisciplinary assessments, interventions, treatments, and outcomes for health-related conditions across a time line

d. A delivery model that brings all services and care providers to clients

e. Established by the U.S. government in 1997 to provide insurance coverage for children of poor and working-class individuals

f. The delivery of individualized nursing care to clients by a team led by a professional nurse

g. Initiated to curtail health care costs in the United States

h. A federal insurance plan to cover adults 65 years of age or older and those with permanent disabilities

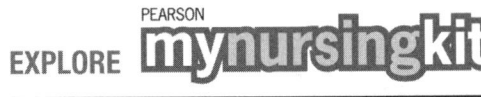

EXPLORE PEARSON mynursingkit

www.mynursingkit.com

MyNursingKit is your one stop for online chapter review materials and resources. Prepare for success with additional NCLEX®-style practice questions, interactive assignments and activities, web links, animations and videos, and more! Register your access code from the front of your textbook at www.mynursingkit.com

Look for these resources:
- NCLEX® Review
- Case Studies
- Videos and Animations

i. The percentage share of an approved charge that is paid by the client

j. A federal public assistance program paid out of general taxes to people who require financial assistance for health care

k. A system in which the best possible use of nursing personnel is based on their educational preparation and resultant skill sets

l. Can be used in concert with other models of nursing delivery

m. Describes a health care system whose goals are to provide cost-effective, quality care that focuses on decreased costs and improved outcomes for groups of clients

n. Group health care agencies that provide health maintenance and treatment services to volunteer enrollees

o. Consists of a group of providers and perhaps a health care agency that provide an insurance company or employer with health services at a discounted rate

KEY TOPIC REVIEW

16. List the three levels of health care services for disease prevention.

17. What are the two primary goals for *Healthy People 2010*?

18. List the four major reasons for the increase in health spending.

19. List five factors affecting health care delivery.

20. List the recommendations for health care reform proposed by *Nursing's Agenda for Health Care Reform* by the ANA (1991) and *Healthy People 2010* by the USDHHS (2000).

21. List the types of home health agencies.

22. What are the major roles for the home health nurse?

23. List some of the needs in the home that the home health nurse assesses to meet the needs of the client and families.

24. List five nursing functions in industrial health care centers.

25. List six services found in large urban hospitals.

26. List five services offered by assisted living centers.

27. List eight of the many potential members of a health care team.

28. List four areas where low income contributes to higher rates of the problem.

CASE STUDY

29. A 36-year-old single mother of four has recently lost her job along with her insurance. She was offered COBRA insurance, but the cost was more than she was receiving in unemployment. Her 7-year-old daughter developed leukemia, which would require expensive medical services. What services will be available to help the family so the daughter will receive the care she needs?

    1. Can social services help her to get an emergency Medicaid card?

    2. With no insurance, will she have to take out a loan?

    3. Can nurses do anything to help with the financial needs of clients?

    4. How do hospitals help when they admit patients without insurance?

REVIEW QUESTIONS

30. The U.S. Department of Health and Human Services contributed to developing *Healthy People 2010*. The main goal of the project is to:

    a. guarantee health coverage for all.

    b. provide money to pay for insurance.

    c. promote national primary prevention for proper nutrition, weight control, exercise, and stress reduction.

    d. increase the number of medical personnel to care for the clients.

31. Hospice nurses work with clients who are dying. They work in homes or facilities. They help to:

    a. provide a diversion to the dying client.

    b. take over for families when they are busy.

    c. supervise the delivery of direct care by other team members.

    d. work only in long-term care facilities.

32. Which of the following age groups is projected to be the fastest growing population in the United States by the year 2020?

    a. Under 20 years

    b. Between 20 and 40 years

    c. Over 85 years

    d. None of the above

33. The elderly population will need many services that will include long-term care facilities. What percent of the elderly are institutionalized?

    a. 30%

    b. 10%

    c. 70%

    d. 5%

34. The lack of medical insurance is directly related to low income, which contributes to which of the following?

    a. More cases of rape, substance abuse, and violence

    b. Higher rates of infectious diseases

    c. Higher deductibles

    d. More use of medical services

35. Payments to individuals with disabilities are made from which of the following?

    a. Social Security

    b. Unemployment Compensation

    c. Supplemental Security Income

    d. Medicaid

36. Private health insurance usually covers about 80% of the cost of health services. How are most of these policies purchased?

    a. Online

    b. Through the mail

    c. At the local hospital

    d. From an employer, union, or student association

37. An insurance that emphasizes client wellness is which of the following?

    a. PHO

    b. HMO

    c. PPO

    d. IDS

38. Nurses help to influence political decision making regarding health care reform by membership in which of the following?

    a. Nursing schools

    b. Professional organizations

    c. Local unions

    d. AARP

39. Which of the following types of health care is directed toward a specific group in a geographic neighborhood?

    a. Planned community health

    b. Traditional health care system

    c. Parish nursing

    d. Community-based health care

40. Videoconferencing allows medical personnel to monitor and receive health information from clients in remote areas. What is it referred to as?

    a. Teladoc

    b. Telepathy

    c. Teleconferencing

    d. Telehealth

41. Which of the following is the most common tool used for interdisciplinary assessments, interventions, treatments, and outcomes for health-related conditions across a time line and has replaced standing orders?

    a. Primary nursing

    b. Patient-focused care

    c. Critical pathways

    d. Differentiated practice

CHAPTER 4

CULTURE AND HERITAGE

KEY TERM REVIEW

Match each term with its appropriate definition.

1. _____ Acculturation
2. _____ Assimilation
3. _____ Bicultural
4. _____ Culturally appropriate
5. _____ Culturally competent
6. _____ Culturally sensitive
7. _____ Culture
8. _____ Culture shock
9. _____ Discrimination
10. _____ Diversity
11. _____ Ethnic
12. _____ Ethnocentrism
13. _____ Folk medicine
14. _____ Heritage
15. _____ Heritage consistency
16. _____ Holistic health
17. _____ Magico-religious health belief
18. _____ Prejudice
19. _____ Scientific health belief

a. Nonphysical traits that are shared by a group of people and passed from generation to generation

b. Something that is handed down from generation to generation

c. Implies that nurses possess some basic knowledge of and constructive attitudes toward the health traditions observed among the diverse cultural groups found in the setting in which they are practicing

d. Implies that nurses possess and apply the underlying background knowledge to provide a given client with the best possible health care

e. Implies that nurses understand and attend to the total context of the client's situation and use a complex combination of knowledge, attitudes, and skills

f. Focuses on providing care within the differences and similarities of the beliefs, values, and patterns of cultures

g. Usually composed of people who have a distinct identity and yet are related to a larger cultural group

h. Used to describe a person who has dual patterns of identification and crosses two cultures, lifestyles, and sets of values

EXPLORE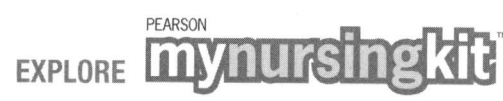

www.mynursingkit.com

MyNursingKit is your one stop for online chapter review materials and resources. Prepare for success with additional NCLEX®-style practice questions, interactive assignments and activities, web links, animations and videos, and more! Register your access code from the front of your textbook at www.mynursingkit.com

Look for these resources:
- NCLEX® Review
- Case Studies
- Videos and Animations

20. _____ Socialization
21. _____ Stereotyping
22. _____ Subculture
23. _____ Transcultural nursing
24. _____ Xenophobia

i. Refers to the fact or state of being different
j. Occurs when people adapt to or borrow traits from another culture
k. The process by which an individual develops a new cultural identity
l. Classification of people according to shared biologic characteristics, genetic markers, or features
m. Negative belief or preference that is generalized about a group and that leads to prejudgment
n. The fear or dislike of people different from oneself
o. Assuming that all members of a culture or ethnic group are alike
p. The belief that one's own culture or way of life is better than that of others
q. The differential treatment of individuals or groups based on categories such as race, ethnicity, gender, social class, or exceptionality
r. Occurs in response to transition from one cultural setting to another
s. A concept developed by Zitzow and Estes (1981), relates to the observance of beliefs and practices of a person's traditional cultural system
t. A complex whole in which each part is related to every other part
u. A group within the social system that claims to possess variable traits such as a common religion or language
v. The process of being raised within a culture and acquiring the characteristics of that group
w. The view that health and illness are controlled by supernatural forces
x. Holds that the forces of nature must be maintained in balance or harmony

KEY TOPIC REVIEW

25. List five things that would be included as part of our culture.

26. List four common issues all groups of people face to be able to adapt to their environment.

27. Give three examples of cultural subgroups.

28. Diversity refers to the fact or state of being different. Name four facts that refer to diversity.

29. List the four various aspects of assimilation.

30. Name four categories of discrimination.

31. In our culturally diversified world, nurses need to be culturally competent and sensitive. List the five constructs developed by Campinha-Bacote's model of cultural competence.

32. List six of the most obvious cultural differences.

33. List five elements included in nonverbal communication.

34. List five things that may be interpreted by a lack of eye contact.

35. List two areas that the implementation of cultural nursing care includes.

36. List eight initiatives for REACH 2010.

CASE STUDY

37. A Russian immigrant was admitted to the hospital with cellulitis to his left leg. He was accompanied by his daughter and 11-year-old grandson. He does not speak English, and the grandson has worked as the interpreter between the physician and the patient. The family is leaving for the evening and you will need to provide his PM care and give him medications. In order to care for the client, you should understand something about his culture and set up a mode of communication.

    1. How can you establish communication without understanding Russian?
    2. What is the best way to provide safe care?
    3. How should you address the client?
    4. How can you explain treatments and medications needed to improve his health?

REVIEW QUESTIONS

38. The United States has at least _____ groups that meet many of the characteristics of an ethnic group.
    a. 25
    b. 50
    c. 78
    d. 106

39. Nurses need strong communication skills and a good understanding of the client's _____ to provide safe and effective care.
    a. heritage
    b. cultural diversity
    c. ethnic heritage
    d. religious beliefs

40. Prior to touching or invading a client's personal space, a nurse must first:
    a. close the door.
    b. ask the family to leave.
    c. introduce him- or herself.
    d. explain the procedure and await permission to proceed.

CHAPTER 4 / Culture and Heritage

41. In order for nurses to understand the cultural background of the client they care for, they should first check into which of the following?

    a. Client's chart

    b. Their own cultural heritage

    c. Health traditions of the client

    d. Client's health practices

42. The United States was known as the melting pot because of all the immigrants. Which of the following is now a more accurate term to describe the way people maintain their cultural heritage?

    a. International heritage

    b. Culturally diverse

    c. Cultural mosaic

    d. Mixed society

43. Health policies and programs were set up to eliminate health disparities for racial and ethnic minority populations. What department established it?

    a. U.S. Department of Justice

    b. U.S. Department of Immigration

    c. U.S. Department for Equality

    d. U.S. Department of Health and Human Services

44. Which agency strives to eliminate racial and ethnic disparities (inequalities) in infant mortality; in screening and management of breast and cervical cancer, cardiovascular diseases, diabetes, and HIV infections/AIDS; and in child and adult immunizations?

    a. REACH

    b. HRSA

    c. GRASP

    d. DHHS

45. As a mobile society we migrate from one geographic area to another, and because each area is different we can go through which of the following?

    a. Stereotyping

    b. Assimilation

    c. Prejudice

    d. Culture shock

46. Human life is one aspect of nature that must be in harmony with the rest of nature, and illness will result when it is not. What is this belief called?

    a. Holistic health

    b. Magico-religious health

    c. Scientific health

    d. Spiritual health

47. Nurses need to learn to be culturally sensitive to the needs of the client. In order to best help the client through the hospital stay, nurses should:

    a. treat all clients the same.

    b. communicate and ask about special needs.

    c. refuse to care for clients that are not American.

    d. provide care only when the client rings for help.

48. How does a nurse provide effective care when a client chooses to follow only cultural practices and declines all prescribed medical or nursing interventions?

    a. Discharge the client since he or she will not accept help offered.

    b. Learn more about the culture and adjust the client goals with the client.

    c. Refuse to care for the client.

    d. Document that the client is noncompliant.

CHAPTER 5

HEALTH BELIEFS AND PRACTICES

KEY TERM REVIEW

Match each term with its appropriate definition.

1. _____ Acupressure
2. _____ Acupuncture
3. _____ Acute
4. _____ Adherence
5. _____ Allopathic
6. _____ Biofeedback
7. _____ Chronic
8. _____ Disease prevention
9. _____ Equilibrium
10. _____ Etiology
11. _____ Health
12. _____ Holism
13. _____ Homeopathy
14. _____ Homeostasis
15. _____ Humanist
16. _____ Hypnosis
17. _____ Naturopathy
18. _____ Remission
19. _____ Risk factors
20. _____ Spirituality

a. State of well-being
b. Concept emphasizing that nurses must keep the whole person in mind
c. Relative constancy of the internal processes of the body
d. Balance, through adaptation to that environment
e. A set of interacting identifiable parts or components
f. Practices that have potentially negative effects on health
g. The extent to which an individual's behavior coincides with medical or health advice
h. Causation of a disease
i. Illness that is typically characterized by severe symptoms of relatively short duration
j. One that lasts for an extended period; can be six months or longer
k. When the symptoms disappear
l. A perspective including propositions such as: the mind and body are indivisible, people have the power to solve their own problems, people are responsible for the patterns of their lives, and well-being is a combination of personal satisfaction and contributions to the larger community

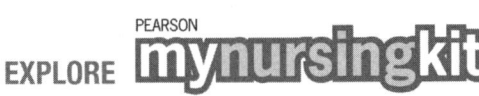

EXPLORE

www.mynursingkit.com

MyNursingKit is your one stop for online chapter review materials and resources. Prepare for success with additional NCLEX®-style practice questions, interactive assignments and activities, web links, animations and videos, and more! Register your access code from the front of your textbook at www.mynursingkit.com

Look for these resources:
- NCLEX® Review
- Case Studies
- Videos and Animations

21. _____ System
22. _____ Wellness

m. Includes the drive to become all that one can be, and is bound to intuition, creativity, and motivation

n. A trance state or an altered state of consciousness in which an individual's concentration is focused and distraction is minimized

o. Method for learned control of physiologic responses of the body

p. System of medicine and way of life with emphasis on client responsibility, client education, health maintenance, and disease prevention

q. Self-healing system assisted by small doses of remedies or medicines used for a variety of acute and chronic disorders

r. Uses needles

s. Uses finger pressure

t. Used to describe Western medical practices

u. State of complete physical, mental, and social well-being, and not merely the absence of disease or infirmity

v. Behavior motivated by a desire to actively avoid illness, detect it early, or maintain functioning within the constraints of illness

KEY TOPIC REVIEW

23. List five areas that are included in the basic aspects of wellness.

24. List the five concepts that describe homeostasis as the relative constancy of the internal processes of the body.

25. List the four main characteristics of homeostatic mechanisms.

26. List Maslow's five human needs.

27. Nurses help clients implement healthy behaviors. List three ways nurses fill that major role.

28. List four things that significantly influence a person's health.

29. List variables that affect people when they are ill.

30. List programs that can be used for the promotion of health.

31. List the concepts of balance for optimal wellness.

32. List Suchman's five stages of illness.

33. List eight areas that encompass a person's total character.

34. List eight things that the nurse explores that impacts a whole person when suffering from the loss of a loved one.

35. List the three steps to the right on the wellness continuum.

36. List the four domains of the inner self.

37. List the elements of the outer system.

CASE STUDY

38. Barb has been working the night shift at the local hospital for more than 10 years. She never takes vacations and claims she needs to work to put her oldest daughter through college and pay medical bills for her son who has leukemia. She has received the nurse of the year award several times and has always been an exemplary nurse. Lately the staff has noticed she has been moody and less than caring for her assigned clients. She is less patient, less tolerant, more irritable, and unhappy. Nurses need to take care of their own needs before they will be effective with others.

   1. What is Barb displaying?

   2. What can her employer do to make her situation more manageable?

   3. How will her clients feel about the care they are receiving?

   4. Nurses should work as a team. Will the other staff members be able to support Barb and help her get back on track?

REVIEW QUESTIONS

39. All living systems require a continuous exchange of energy. These systems are in a constant state of which of the following?

    a. Homeostasis

    b. Repair

    c. Change

    d. Negative feedback

40. What is one of the most useful strategies for raising the level of knowledge and awareness of individuals and groups about health habits?

    a. Role playing

    b. Information dissemination

    c. Reading

    d. Education

41. Which of the following is a state of focused attention that encourages changes in attitudes, behavior, and physiologic reactions?

    a. Hypnosis

    b. Hypnotherapy

    c. Meditation

    d. Guided imagery

42. The use of water as a healing treatment is used to decrease pain, decrease fever, reduce swelling, reduce cramps, induce sleep, and improve physical and mental tone. What is this called?

    a. Hydrotherapy

    b. Hydroplaning

    c. Water boarding

    d. Hypnotherapy

43. Nurses not only care for clients when they are sick, they also help teach clients to avoid the development of disease in the future and of all the interventions to limit progression of a disease process. What is this called?

    a. Medical care contact

    b. Health promotion

    c. Impact on the client

    d. Health protection

44. Employers who offer health-focused programs have benefits for the employees and employers by helping to control the rising cost of health care and to reduce which of the following?

    a. Overtime

    b. Coinsurance payments

    c. Attrition

    d. Employee absenteeism

45. In which stage does a person acknowledge having a problem, seriously consider changing a specific behavior, actively gather information, and verbalize plans to change the behavior in the near future?

    a. Precontemplation stage

    b. Preparation stage

    c. Contemplation stage

    d. Action stage

46. What stage occurs when the person actively implements behavioral and cognitive strategies and plans to interrupt previous health risk behaviors and adopt new ones? This stage requires the greatest commitment of time and energy.

    a. Action stage

    b. Contemplation stage

    c. Precontemplation stage

    d. Maintenance stage

47. What stage has the ultimate goal where the individual has complete confidence that the problem is no longer a temptation or threat?

    a. Contemplation stage

    b. Action stage

    c. Termination stage

    d. Maintenance stage

48. Name the basic tool for a nurse in a health promotion role that emphasizes teaching the client self-care responsibility.

    a. Planning

    b. Nursing process

    c. Assessment

    d. Evaluation

49. How can the nurse's knowledge of developmental stage theories be used?

    a. To help educate the client

    b. In parental and client education, counseling, and anticipatory guidance

    c. To develop a nursing care plan

    d. To promote the theories of a given theorist

50. What can health belief models do?

    a. Help determine whether an individual will participate in disease prevention and health promotion activities

    b. Provide useful tools in developing programs for helping people live healthier lifestyles

    c. Develop a more positive attitude toward preventive health measures

    d. Have a major influence over health care

CHAPTER 6

CRITICAL THINKING AND CLINICAL REASONING

KEY TERM REVIEW

Match each term with its appropriate definition.

1. _____ Accuracy
2. _____ Assumption
3. _____ Clarity
4. _____ Clinical judgment
5. _____ Clinical reasoning
6. _____ Concept
7. _____ Conclusion
8. _____ Creativity
9. _____ Critical analysis
10. _____ Critical thinking
11. _____ Decision making
12. _____ Deductive reasoning
13. _____ Implication
14. _____ Inductive reasoning
15. _____ Inference
16. _____ Intellectual standard
17. _____ Interpretation
18. _____ Intuition
19. _____ Logic (or logical)
20. _____ Precision
21. _____ Reasoning

a. Reflective reasoning process that guides a nurse in generating, implementing, and evaluating approaches for dealing with client care and professional concerns

b. Thinking that results in the development of new ideas and products

c. Differentiating facts from opinions

d. Application of a set of questions to a particular situation or idea to determine essential information and ideas and discard superfluous information and ideas

e. Generalizations that are formed from a set of facts or observations

f. Reasoning from the general premise to the specific conclusion

g. Understanding or learning of things without the conscious use of reasoning

h. Critical-thinking process for choosing the best actions to meet a desired goal

i. An active process by which nurses make judgments

j. Conclusions and opinions about clients' health drawn from patient data

k. Process that guides a nurse in generating, implementing, and evaluating approaches for dealing with client care and professional concerns

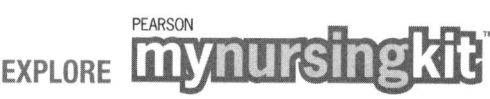

www.mynursingkit.com

MyNursingKit is your one stop for online chapter review materials and resources. Prepare for success with additional NCLEX®-style practice questions, interactive assignments and activities, web links, animations and videos, and more! Register your access code from the front of your textbook at www.mynursingkit.com

Look for these resources:
- NCLEX® Review
- Case Studies
- Videos and Animations

22. _____ Relevance
23. _____ Significance

l. Exactness or accuracy

m. Indirect suggestion

n. Ability to avoid errors

o. Decision based on facts

p. Clearness of expression

q. Establish a meaning

r. Something taken for granted

s. Understanding or grasp

t. Importance of having great meaning

u. Abstract thinking

v. Theory of reasoning

w. Importance

KEY TOPIC REVIEW

24. Creative thinkers must have knowledge of the problem, and they use what they know to help solve problems. List three things that help nurses generate ideas.

25. List four ways nurses use critical thinking.

26. Name three interrelated processes that promote creativity to enhance the end result.

27. List three complex mental processes that use cognitive critical-thinking skills.

28. List the phases of the nursing process.

29. List the five points employed in Socratic questioning.

30. List nine traits that a critical thinker works to develop.

31. List sequential steps for decision making.

32. List five areas that nurses must embrace to gain insight by exploring perspectives of persons who will actively create a stimulating environment encouraging differences of opinion and a fair examination of ideas and options.

33. List five things that nurses accomplish by being creative.

34. List the core attributes of critical thinking.

35. List four things nurses do when faced with several client needs at the same time.

36. List seven requirements for effective clinical reasoning and decision making.

CASE STUDY

37. Critical-thinking skills need to be developed over time. Graduate nurses starting their first jobs have an orientation period to work with veteran nurses who hopefully will guide them to develop the best clinical decisions.

    1. What can graduate nurses do to acquire these skills?

    2. How can the orienting nurse ensure the graduate nurse is developing critical-thinking skills?

    3. Nurses work together as a team. Can we develop a better way to approach health care decisions?

    4. Are student nurses instructed in the importance of using critical-thinking skills?

REVIEW QUESTIONS

38. What is the method of questioning used in critical analysis by a Greek philosopher?

    a. Aristotle

    b. Plato

    c. Socratic

    d. Heraclitus

39. The nursing process has many dimensions, and nurses continuously must interpret client data and come to a conclusion that will best help the client. These decisions can mean either taking or not taking action. What does clinical reasoning begin with?

    a. Narrative thinking

    b. Clinical judgment

    c. Analytic processes

    d. Cognitive skills

40. Technology is growing exponentially in the medical field and affecting how nurses care for clients. When an alarm sounds on a machine or piece of equipment, what must nurses remember to do first?

    a. Check the machine.

    b. Check the electrical outlets.

    c. Check the client.

    d. Just ignore it.

41. Student nurses grow as they go through clinical experiences. It is the opportunity to use what is learned in the classroom and put it into action. One of the many responsibilities that instructors have is to give constructive criticism to help students improve their abilities. What is the first key to clinical success?

    a. Responsibility

    b. Accountability

    c. Professionalism

    d. Safety

42. Along with the responsibility of caring for clients also come honesty, ethical behavior, and good morals. Nurses and students should always admit their errors. If a medication error occurs and is not reported, it could cause irreversible damage. If the error is reported, counteractive measures can be taken. What is this called?

    a. Responsibility

    b. Accountability

    c. Professionalism

    d. Safety

43. Thought processes used by nurses have many areas to cover, and nurses use experience and knowledge to put together solutions that will help the client's recovery. What types of thinkers are able to build on their knowledge and develop a solution?

   a. Creative

   b. Decision makers

   c. Advanced

   d. Critical

44. Nursing schools require many courses to diversify and build on. The basic knowledge helps to give a good foundation for which of the following?

   a. Inductive reasoning

   b. Decision making

   c. Creative thinking

   d. Critical thinking

45. Nurses care for many clients with diverse and multiple health issues. When using critical-thinking skills to figure out one issue, nurses can apply the knowledge to another client with similar health issues. Common approaches include trial and error, intuition, research, and science. In obtaining information and developing solutions, what is this called?

   a. Deductive reasoning

   b. Inductive reasoning

   c. Problem solving

   d. Decision making

46. What is the Mind Map for Critical Thinking in Nursing?

   a. A concept map of directions for the nursing process

   b. A map used to determine if the current course of action is the best one

   c. A visual depiction of the interactive loops of concepts used in critical thinking

   d. A map used to improve future actions

47. What happens to nurses who do not participate in continuing education?

   a. They lose their nursing skills.

   b. They do not get raises.

   c. They will need to go back to school.

   d. They become dangerous care providers.

48. What are interpersonal skills?

   a. Skills developed to get along with other people

   b. Skills that improve relationships between the nurse and others

   c. Internal skills everyone possesses

   d. Skills that have to be learned from another person

CHAPTER 7

THE NURSING PROCESS

KEY TERM REVIEW

Match each term with its appropriate definition.

1. _____ Assessing
2. _____ Cephalocaudal
3. _____ Collaborative care plan
4. _____ Concept map
5. _____ Cues
6. _____ Data
7. _____ Defining characteristics
8. _____ Desired outcomes
9. _____ Diagnosis
10. _____ Discharge planning
11. _____ Evaluating
12. _____ Evaluation statement
13. _____ Goals
14. _____ Implementing
15. _____ Indicator
16. _____ Individualized care plan
17. _____ Interview
18. _____ Nursing diagnosis

a. Planned communication or conversation with a purpose

b. The act of "double-checking" or verifying data to confirm that it is accurate and factual

c. A statement or conclusion regarding the nature of a phenomenon

d. A clinical judgment about individual, family, or community responses to actual and potential health problems/life processes

e. A classification system or set of categories arranged based on a single principle or set of principles

f. The systematic and continuous collection, organization, validation, and documentation of data

g. Tailored to meet the unique needs of a specific client—needs that are not addressed by the standardized plan

h. A visual tool in which ideas or data are enclosed in circles or boxes of some shape and relationships between these are indicated by connecting lines or arrows

i. The cluster of signs and symptoms that indicate the presence of a particular diagnostic label

EXPLORE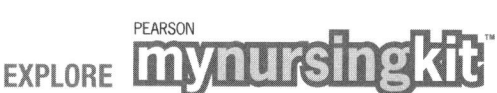

www.mynursingkit.com

MyNursingKit is your one stop for online chapter review materials and resources. Prepare for success with additional NCLEX®-style practice questions, interactive assignments and activities, web links, animations and videos, and more! Register your access code from the front of your textbook at www.mynursingkit.com

Look for these resources:
- NCLEX® Review
- Case Studies
- Videos and Animations

29

19. _____ Planning
20. _____ Priority setting
21. _____ Procedures
22. _____ Protocol
23. _____ Quality improvement
24. _____ Taxonomy
25. _____ Validation

j. The process of establishing a preferential sequence for addressing nursing diagnoses and interventions

k. A deliberative, systematic phase of the nursing process that involves decision making and problem solving

l. The process of anticipating and planning for needs after discharge

m. A more concrete individual, family, or community state, behavior, or perception that serves as a cue for measuring an outcome

n. A planned, ongoing, purposeful activity in which clients and health care professionals determine (a) the client's progress toward achievement of goals/outcomes and (b) the effectiveness of the nursing care plan

o. Consists of two parts: a conclusion and supporting data

p. Internal assessment by health care providers and increasing awareness by the public that medical errors are not uncommon and can be lethal

q. Consists of doing and documenting the activities that are specific nursing actions needed to carry out the interventions

r. Head-to-toe approach beginning the examination at the head; progressing to the neck, thorax, abdomen, and extremities; and ending at the toes

s. Information

t. Subjective or objective data that can be directly observed by the nurse

u. Actions commonly required for a particular group of clients

v. Specify what is to be done in a given situation

w. Standardized plan that outlines the care required for clients with common, predictable conditions

x. Broad statements about the client's status and desired outcomes

y. A five-point scale (a measure) that is used to rate the client's status on each indicator

KEY TOPIC REVIEW

26. List the five phases of the nursing process.

27. List the four different types of assessment.

28. List the five client's perceived needs.

29. List the four closely related activities for the assessment process.

30. List the types of information found in the database about a client.

31. List six things that are included in subjective data.

32. List the three principal methods used to collect data.

33. List the five types of nursing diagnoses.

34. List five reasons for a client not to provide accurate subjective data.

35. List four things that medical records can provide about a client's present and past health and illness patterns.

36. List five purposes for a planned interview.

37. List four things that can influence an interview.

38. List the four techniques that the nurse uses to perform a physical examination.

39. List in order the progression of the cephalocaudal physical examination.

40. List Roy's observable behavior adaptation model that is classified into four categories.

CASE STUDY

41. John Smith is a 36-year-old who was admitted to the hospital on the medical–surgical unit. He has been a paraplegic for five years as a result of an industrial accident. He uses a manual wheelchair and lives alone in a handicap accessible apartment. He was admitted for recurrent decubiti on his coccyx area. The nurse noted during the admission process that the client had a strong body odor from poor hygiene, including a strong urine odor. She also noted his wheelchair was extremely soiled with food crumbs and dirt. He was scheduled for surgery the next morning.

    1. What are the important goals the nurse needs to accomplish to assist the client?
    2. What independent and collaborative interventions can the nurse provide?
    3. What direct or indirect care can be offered to John?
    4. What nursing diagnosis would be used on his care plan?

REVIEW QUESTIONS

42. All clients admitted to a hospital need to have an initial assessment consisting of a history and physical performed and documented within 24 hours of admission. This rule was mandated by what organization?

    a. American Nursing Association
    b. North American Nursing Diagnosis Association
    c. American Association for Retired People
    d. Joint Commission on Accreditation of Healthcare Organizations

43. Ralph was brought into the emergency department with chest pain, blurred vision, and an unsteady gait. Using the nursing process, what should the nurse do first?

    a. Plan
    b. Implement
    c. Assess
    d. Evaluate

44. Communication skills are vital to the nurse–client relationship. What level of communication do nurses use?

    a. Nonverbal

    b. Social

    c. Structured

    d. Therapeutic

45. Nurses perform technical skills working with equipment, giving injections, changing dressings, lifting, and repositioning clients. These skills are known as which of the following?

    a. Psychiatric

    b. Psychomotor

    c. Psychologic

    d. Physiologic

46. The last phase of the nursing process is an important aspect since conclusions drawn from this phase will help to determine if further assessment is indicated. What is the last phase?

    a. Implementing

    b. Diagnosing

    c. Planning

    d. Evaluation

47. Which phases in the nursing process overlap?

    a. Evaluating and assessing

    b. Evaluating and planning

    c. Evaluating and implementing

    d. Implementing and planning

48. During what step does the nurse identify the desired outcomes (indicators) that will be used to measure client goal achievement?

    a. Implementing

    b. Assessing

    c. Planning

    d. Diagnosing

49. The conclusion and supporting data help to form which statement?

    a. Assessment

    b. Implementation

    c. Planning

    d. Evaluation

50. Nurses are also involved in evaluating and modifying the overall quality of care given to groups of clients. What is this an essential part of?

    a. Professional accountability

    b. Quality assurance

    c. Quality improvement

    d. Professional responsibility

51. Nurses use problem-solving skills to identify a client's health status and actual or potential health problems and needs. What organized approach is used?

    a. Implementing

    b. Nursing process

    c. Assessing

    d. Diagnosing

52. What is the difference between objective and subjective data?

    a. Subjective is what the client tells you, and objective is what you can see.

    b. Subjective is what you see, and objective is what you are told by the client.

    c. Subjective is the client's diagnosis, and objective is what you see in the chart.

    d. Subjective is what the doctor sees, and objective is what the nurse sees.

53. When does effective discharge planning begin?

    a. When the physician writes the orders

    b. 24 hours before the client goes home

    c. During the first client contact

    d. When the client is ready

54. What is a holistic individualized plan of care?

    a. A plan that will meet the client's unique needs

    b. A plan in which nurses use the client's nursing diagnoses to develop goals and nursing interventions

    c. A care plan that addresses all the needs of the client

    d. A plan that nurses promote for the whole person

55. Nurses are responsible to assess clients and develop care plans that address existing and potential problems, but what type of interventions are appropriate when a client has no health problems?

    a. Prevention interventions

    b. Health promotion interventions

    c. Treatments

    d. Observations

CHAPTER 8

INFORMATICS, DOCUMENTATION, AND REPORTING

KEY TERM REVIEW

Match each term with its appropriate definition.

1. _____ Charting
2. _____ Client record
3. _____ Computer-based patient records
4. _____ Documenting
5. _____ Electronic medical record (EMR)
6. _____ Flow sheet
7. _____ Focus charting
8. _____ Hardware
9. _____ Hospital information system
10. _____ Kardex
11. _____ Narrative charting
12. _____ Nursing informatics
13. _____ Peripherals
14. _____ PIE
15. _____ Problem-oriented record
16. _____ Progress note
17. _____ Report

a. Oral, written, or computer-based communication intended to convey information to others

b. Process of making an entry on a client record

c. Problems, interventions, evaluation model

d. Formal, legal document that provides evidence of a client's care

e. Traditional client record

f. Acronym for subjective data, objective data, assessment, and planning

g. A deviation to what is planned on the critical pathway

h. Uses specific assessment criteria in a particular format, such as human needs or functional health patterns

i. Client's progress in relation to the goals or outcomes defined in the plan of care

j. Intended to make the client, and client concerns and strengths, the focus of care

k. Concise method of organizing and recording data about a client

l. The power supply, disk drives, chips, and connections for all the other computer hardware

18. _____ SOAP
19. _____ Source-oriented record
20. _____ Variance

m. An MIS that focuses on the types of data needed to manage client care activities and health care organizations

n. The science of using computer information systems in the practice of nursing

o. A traditional part of the source-oriented record

p. Electronic client data retrieval by caregivers, administrators, accreditors, and other persons who require the data

q. Arrangement of data according to the problems the client has rather than the source of the information

r. The actual components of the computer that allow them to function

s. A formal piece of writing that contains information

t. Permit electronic client data retrieval by caregivers, administrators, accreditors, and other persons who require the data

KEY TOPIC REVIEW

21. List five purposes for which client records are kept.

22. List the five requirements for client record documentation from the Joint Commission on Accreditation of Healthcare Organizations (JCAHO).

23. List the four items that a client's record can provide for educational purposes.

24. List six documentation systems that are in current use.

25. List the four basic components of the POMR.

26. Name the items in the acronym SOAP.

27. List the nine areas addressed on the nursing care summary for clients in a long-term care facility.

28. List the two most common computer systems used by nurses.

29. List the ways computers are used in the health care system.

30. List five forms of information that can be completed at the bedside with computerized bedside data entry systems.

31. Identify four ways the EMR could improve health care as stated by the Computer-Based Patient Record Institute.

32. List the information that would commonly be included in a telephone report.

33. Name the items in the acronym PIE.

34. List five items JCAHO requires that the clinical record should include.

35. List three things the OBRA law requires.

36. List three services for which Medicare provides reimbursement for clients in a long-term care facility.

CHAPTER 8 / Informatics, Documentation, and Reporting

CASE STUDY

37. Judy was called in to work the night shift. Her unit was short staffed and several practical nurses were pulled to cover the busy medical–surgical unit. Since Judy was only one of three RNs on the shift, the work was divided and each RN was responsible to do the charting for the PNs. After working a 12-hour shift and charting on 14 clients, she realized she had documented two charts on the wrong client. She was too tired to stay and correct the chart and thought she could do it when she came back in on her next shift. That day one client was discharged and the chart went to medical records, and one client was transferred to a long-term care facility and copies of the chart were sent with him.

   1. What should she do about the charts?
   2. How should the corrections be made?
   3. Was being tired an acceptable excuse not to correct the charts?
   4. What are some legal ramifications of having the wrong documentation in a client's chart?

REVIEW QUESTIONS

38. The client's clinical record must have accurate and complete documentation with codable diagnoses to support all charges in order to receive payments from which of the following?

    a. Medicare
    b. Client
    c. Facility
    d. Provider

39. What charting system provides a holistic perspective of the client and the client's needs as well as providing a nursing process framework for the progress notes?

    a. Charting by exception
    b. Focus charting
    c. SOAP charting
    d. PIE charting

40. What model uses a multidisciplinary approach to planning and documenting client care, using critical pathways?

    a. Charting by exception
    b. PIE charting
    c. Focus charting
    d. Case management

41. What charting system alerts the nurse to any changes in the client's condition?

    a. Focus charting
    b. SOAP
    c. Charting by exception
    d. PIE

42. What model is cost effective and uses a multidisciplinary approach to planning and documenting with the use of critical pathways?

    a. Charting by exception

    b. Case management

    c. SOAP

    d. Focus charting

43. Jody finished her documentation for her six clients. As she was checking her work, she realized she had written a client assessment on the wrong chart. What should she do?

    a. Use white correction fluid.

    b. Draw squiggly lines through it.

    c. Draw a line and write "error" above it.

    d. Draw a line and write "mistaken entry" above it.

44. The use of technology has created more problems with the privacy act, and HIPAA continues to make changes to ensure client confidentiality. What should faxed material have to help keep the information private?

    a. Name of the recipient

    b. Name of the sender

    c. Cover sheet with instruction to destroy the information if it was received erroneously

    d. Return address and fax number

45. Nurses need to protect themselves from malpractice by using what steps and framework?

    a. Nursing care plan

    b. NANDA

    c. Charting by exception

    d. Nursing process

46. Nurses can use a handheld device that can send information on a client to PCs, networks, or phone systems. The device can also be used for data entry and retrieval devices. What is it called?

    a. Blackberry

    b. Cell phone

    c. Personal digital assistant (PDA)

    d. Computer

47. What organization set up a code of ethics that states that ". . . the nurse has a duty to maintain confidentiality of all patient information"?

    a. OBRA

    b. JCAHO

    c. HIPAA

    d. ANA

48. What is the PIE system disadvantage?

    a. It eliminates the traditional care plan.

    b. It incorporates an ongoing care plan into the progress notes.

    c. The nurse must review all the nursing notes.

    d. The nurse must determine which problems are current.

49. What does the case management model incorporate along with critical pathways?

    a. Graphics and flow sheets

    b. Chart and calendars

    c. Checks and balances

    d. Collaboration and teamwork

CHAPTER 9

PROMOTING HEALTH THROUGHOUT THE LIFESPAN

KEY TERM REVIEW

Match each term with its appropriate definition.

1. _____ Accommodation
2. _____ Adaptation
3. _____ Assimilation
4. _____ Baby boomer
5. _____ Defense mechanism
6. _____ Denver Developmental Screening Test
7. _____ Development
8. _____ Developmental stage
9. _____ Developmental task
10. _____ Failure to thrive
11. _____ Generation X
12. _____ Generation Y
13. _____ Growth
14. _____ Menopause
15. _____ Morality
16. _____ Peer
17. _____ Personality
18. _____ Primary sexual characteristics

a. Scale used to assess the developmental, intellectual, motor, and social maturity of children from birth to age 9

b. Group identified as being principled, idealistic, experts, caring, savvy, and diverse

c. Process of change whereby cognitive processes mature sufficiently to allow the person to solve problems that were unsolvable before

d. Increase in the complexity of function and skill progression

e. Task that arises at or about a certain period in the life of an individual, successful achievement of which leads to happiness and to success with later tasks, while failure leads to unhappiness in the individual, disapproval by society, and difficulty with later tasks

f. A unique syndrome in which an infant falls below the fifth percentile for height and weight on a standard growth chart or is falling in percentiles on a growth chart

g. A group of those born in or after 1980; perceive themselves as idealistic

h. Someone who is the equal of somebody else, e.g., in age or social class

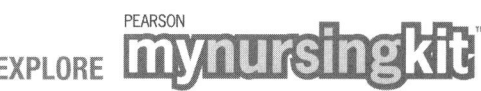

EXPLORE mynursingkit

www.mynursingkit.com

MyNursingKit is your one stop for online chapter review materials and resources. Prepare for success with additional NCLEX®-style practice questions, interactive assignments and activities, web links, animations and videos, and more! Register your access code from the front of your textbook at www.mynursingkit.com

Look for these resources:
- NCLEX® Review
- Case Studies
- Videos and Animations

19. _____ Puberty
20. _____ Regression
21. _____ Repression
22. _____ Secondary sexual characteristics
23. _____ Self-concept
24. _____ Separation anxiety

i. The cessation of menstruation, occurring when 12 months pass without a menstrual period

j. The requirements necessary for people to live together in a society

k. Describes the physical changes such as an increase in size; includes height, weight, bone size, and dentition

l. Theory proposing that life is a sequence of levels of achievement, each stage signaling a task that must be accomplished

m. A complex concept that is difficult to define, can be considered as the outward (interpersonal) expression of the inner (intrapersonal) self

n. Reverting to an earlier development stage, which may be indicated by bed-wetting or using baby talk

o. The fear and frustration that comes with parental separation

p. Related to the organs necessary for reproduction

q. A culmination of body image development, feelings about self, adaptive and defensive mechanisms, reactions from others, and one's perceptions of these reactions, attitudes, values, and many of life's experiences

r. The process of removing experiences, thoughts, and impulses from awareness

s. A generation of people born roughly during the years 1965 to 1980 in Western countries; often regarded as disillusioned, cynical, or apathetic

t. Coping behavior giving the ability to handle the demands made by the environment

u. The result of conflicts between the id's impulses and the anxiety created by the conflicts due to social and environmental restrictions

v. The first stage of adolescence, starting between ages 10–14 in girls and 12–16 in boys; defined by sexual organs beginning to grow and mature

w. The process through which humans encounter and react to new situations by using the mechanisms they already possess

x. Differentiation between the male from the female but does not relate to reproduction

KEY TOPIC REVIEW

25. List four growth measurements that include indicators of physiologic growth.

26. Development is the behavioral changes associated with aging. List four things it includes.

27. List seven factors that influence growth and development.

28. List five concepts that were introduced about development by Sigmund Freud.

29. List Erikson's eight stages of development.

30. List Freud's stages of psychosexual development.

31. List the five major phases of Piaget's cognitive developmental process.

32. List four adaptive mechanisms.

33. List the four leading causes of death in the 10 to 24 age group.

34. List five theorists that were discussed in the chapter.

35. List three needs that parents and caregivers should meet to enhance a sense of trust in infants.

36. List the specific components of growth and development that the theorists considered.

37. List eight concepts that encompass a person's personality.

38. Identify nine temperamental qualities as seen in children's behavior.

CASE STUDY

39. Jesse's 5-year-old daughter Melanie suffered tonsillitis for three years, so the pediatric physician decided to have her tonsils removed. After the surgery Melanie started wetting the bed and would not leave her mother's side. She regressed to a younger time in her life because of trauma caused by the surgery.

    1. What stage of Erikson's should she be in at age 5?
    2. What stage has she regressed to?
    3. What can her mother do to promote her return to the stage she should be in?
    4. Will surgery or traumas always cause clients to regress to another stage of development?

REVIEW QUESTIONS

40. What is the realistic part of the person's mind balancing the gratification demands of the id with the limitations of social and physical circumstances?

    a. Id
    b. Ego
    c. Superego
    d. Defense mechanisms

41. Nurses need to have an understanding of the stages of development from birth to death. These developmental stages are influential in coping with stresses. They were proposed by which theorist?

    a. Freud
    b. Erikson
    c. Piaget
    d. Havighurst

CHAPTER 9 / Promoting Health Throughout the Lifespan

42. These developmental stages follow a sequence where each stage has a task that must be accomplished before moving on to the next level or it can damage the level. What theorist developed these stages?

    a. Piaget

    b. Freud

    c. Havighurst

    d. Erikson

43. What theorist wrote "a task which arises at or about a certain period in the life of an individual, successful achievement of which leads to his happiness and to success with later tasks, while failure leads to unhappiness in the individual, disapproval by society, and difficulty with later tasks"?

    a. Erikson

    b. Havighurst

    c. Freud

    d. Piaget

44. What theorist believes that although physical capabilities and functions decrease with old age, mental and social capacities tend to increase in the latter part of life?

    a. Vygotsky

    b. Havighurst

    c. Peck

    d. Freud

45. Which theorist wrote that cognitive development is an orderly, sequential process in which a variety of new experiences (stimuli) must exist before intellectual abilities can develop?

    a. Gould

    b. Kohlberg

    c. Freud

    d. Piaget

46. What is it called when an infant falls below the fifth percentile for weight and height on a standard growth chart or is falling in percentiles on a growth chart?

    a. Failure to thrive

    b. Infant colic

    c. Separation anxiety

    d. Regression

47. What are the methods the ego uses to fulfill the needs of the id?

    a. Defense mechanisms

    b. Character traits

    c. Behaviors

    d. Self-esteem

48. What is Freud's psychosexual stage that begins in puberty and continues through the rest of the lifespan?

    a. Oral stage

    b. Pregenital stage

    c. Genital stage

    d. Anal stage

49. What theorist believed that learning is basic to life and that people continue to learn throughout the lifespan?

    a. Havighurst

    b. Freud

    c. Piaget

    d. Skinner

50. What needs do infants depend on adults for during their first year of life?

    a. Financial support

    b. Nutrition and love

    c. Safety and warmth

    d. Physiologic and psychologic needs

51. What did Freud call his proposal of the underlying motivation to human development that is dynamic, psychic energy?

    a. Libido

    b. Ego

    c. Id

    d. Superego

52. Nurses need to have an understanding of Erikson's developmental stages so they can promote the positive resolution of a developmental task by which of the following?

    a. Changing the outcome if the developmental stages are not met

    b. Working with the client to accomplish the task for better health

    c. Providing the individual with appropriate opportunities and encouragement

    d. Explaining the developmental stages

53. What was Kohlberg's highest level for moral development?

    a. Moral turpitude

    b. Moral reasoning

    c. Moral findings

    d. Moral domination

CHAPTER 10

PROMOTING HEALTH IN ELDERS

KEY TERM REVIEW

Match each term with its appropriate definition.

1. _____ Adult day care
2. _____ Ageism
3. _____ Assisted living
4. _____ Continuity theory
5. _____ Dementia
6. _____ Disengagement theory
7. _____ Geriatrics
8. _____ Gerontology
9. _____ Long-term memory
10. _____ Perception
11. _____ Recent memory
12. _____ Sensory memory
13. _____ Short-term memory

a. A medical term associated with the medical care of an older adult (e.g., diseases and disabilities)

b. The ability to interpret the environment depending on the acuteness of the senses

c. The progressive loss of cognitive function

d. A focus on social activities or health care where the level of nursing care can vary (e.g., bathing, medical administration, wound dressings)

e. Remembering information for a brief time regarding activities within a short time to a few hours

f. The repository for information stored for periods longer than 72 hours and usually weeks and years

g. The deep and profound prejudice in American society against older adults

h. Momentary perception of stimuli from the environment

i. An option for older adults who do not feel safe living alone or require additional help with activities on a daily basis

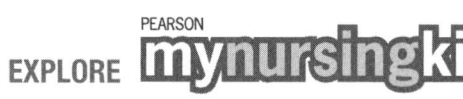

EXPLORE mynursingkit

www.mynursingkit.com

MyNursingKit is your one stop for online chapter review materials and resources. Prepare for success with additional NCLEX®-style practice questions, interactive assignments and activities, web links, animations and videos, and more! Register your access code from the front of your textbook at www.mynursingkit.com

Look for these resources:
- NCLEX® Review
- Case Studies
- Videos and Animations

j. Storage of information held in the brain for immediate use or what one has in mind at the moment

k. The study of aging from a biologic, psychologic, and sociologic perspective

l. The theory that people maintain their values, habits, and behavior in old age

m. Aging that involves mutual withdrawal between the older person and others in the person's environment

KEY TOPIC REVIEW

14. List five roles for the gerontological nurse.

15. Hospice nurses are specially trained to meet the needs of the older population. List five areas that they need to have a good understanding of.

16. List four settings where rehabilitation for the elderly can be found.

17. List three theories for explaining physical aging.

18. List the physical changes that occur as a body ages.

19. List five factors that can help to reduce the risk of cardiovascular disease in the elderly.

20. List six foods that should be avoided that can irritate the bladder of an older person.

21. What are some things that grandparents contribute to their families besides gifts and money? List four things.

22. List five major reasons for grandparents raising grandchildren.

23. List four things contained in intellectual capacity.

24. List five things that influence the nurse's values that should be identified especially in caring for the elderly client.

25. List three reasons why people are living longer.

26. List five socioeconomic characteristics that may differ between the young-old and old-old groups.

27. List three modifiable risk factors that the gerontological nurse often focuses on when teaching the elderly.

CASE STUDY

28. Anabelle is 82 years old and lives alone in her own home. She has been a widow for four years and has still not gotten used to living alone. She has two daughters and a son but they all live in different states. Lately she has not felt like going grocery shopping or cooking for herself and as a result she has lost weight. She has a car but can only drive during the daytime. Most of her friends have died or are in long-term care facilities.

    1. What services are available to her so that she can stay in her own home?

    2. Can her problems be due to a medical condition?

    3. Do we judge all elderly people the same and see a pattern with the aging process?

    4. Would she be better going into a retirement home or living with her adult children in another state?

REVIEW QUESTIONS

29. One of the socioeconomic facts is that those with a higher education will also have which of the following?

    a. Double the income

    b. No change in income

    c. Higher income

    d. Lower income

30. As people age, they lose the ability to hear and they experience loss of visual acuity. What is the term used for loss of hearing?

    a. Presbyopia

    b. Presbycusis

    c. Presbyterian

    d. Presbyacuity

31. What theorist hypothesized that an older person at the preconventional level obeys rules to avoid pain and the displeasure of others?

    a. Freud

    b. Skinner

    c. Kohlberg

    d. Piaget

32. What theorist developed a theory of moral reasoning based on the concept of caring and that women do not follow Kohlberg's theory?

    a. Gilligan

    b. Skinner

    c. Piaget

    d. Pratt

33. Elder abuse is on the rise, especially with the poor economy. When nurses or medical professionals suspect a family member of abusing or being abused, what should they do?

    a. Ignore it.

    b. Report it.

    c. Discuss it with the client.

    d. Accuse the family of abuse.

34. What is the most common type of dementia, which is suffered by the elderly but can affect adults in their 30s?

    a. Organic brain disorder

    b. Alzheimer's disease

    c. Intracranial pressure

    d. Normal pressure hydrocephalus

35. Many older adults take their faith and religious practice very seriously, and display a high level of which of the following?

    a. Alcoholism

    b. Tithing

    c. Attending church functions

    d. Spirituality

36. Which of the following are the primary users of health care services from acute care facilities to rehabilitation, long-term care, and the community?

    a. Young adults

    b. Middle-aged adults

    c. Older adults

    d. Teens

37. What is the objective of long-term care?

    a. To keep older folks off the street

    b. To provide the same opportunities to everyone in that age group

    c. To relieve their children of having to care for them

    d. To provide a place of safety and care to attain optimal wellness and independence for each individual

38. What do age-related changes result in due to the decreased mobility and safety of the older adult?

    a. At risk for falls and fractures

    b. At risk for higher insurance premiums

    c. At risk for longer hospital stays

    d. At risk for limited social activities

39. The excretory function of the kidney diminishes with age, decreasing the kidney's filtering abilities which can also create problems with medications. What should the nurse look out for?

    a. Signs of toxicity

    b. Medications that are excreted through the kidneys

    c. Medications that are excreted through the liver

    d. Drugs that are metabolized in the kidney

40. What is the major age-related change in sexual response in both older men and women?

    a. Low sperm count

    b. Decreased libido

    c. Decrease in hormones

    d. Timing

41. How do older people who attain ego integrity view life?

    a. They view it as an acceptable completion of life.

    b. They wish they could live life over.

    c. They view life with a sense of wholeness and derive satisfaction from past accomplishments.

    d. They believe they have made poor choices during life.

CHAPTER 11

PROMOTING HEALTH IN THE FAMILY

KEY TERM REVIEW

Match each term with its appropriate definition.

1. _____ Extended family
2. _____ Family
3. _____ Family-centered nursing
4. _____ Negative feedback
5. _____ Nuclear family
6. _____ Positive feedback
7. _____ Subsystem
8. _____ Suprasystem
9. _____ System

a. A family structure of parents and their offspring
b. A component of a complex system
c. Looking back up the hierarchy, the system above other systems
d. Influences behavior and stimulates change
e. Influences behavior and inhibits change
f. Nursing that considers the health of the family as a unit, in addition to the health of the individual
g. A basic unit of society consisting of those individuals, male or female, youth or adult, legally or not legally related, genetically or not genetically related, who are considered by the others to represent their significant persons
h. A set of interacting identifiable parts or components
i. The relatives of nuclear families, such as grandparents, aunts, or uncles

EXPLORE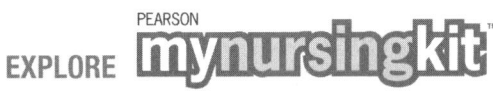

www.mynursingkit.com

MyNursingKit is your one stop for online chapter review materials and resources. Prepare for success with additional NCLEX®-style practice questions, interactive assignments and activities, web links, animations and videos, and more! Register your access code from the front of your textbook at www.mynursingkit.com

Look for these resources:
- NCLEX® Review
- Case Studies
- Videos and Animations

KEY TOPIC REVIEW

10. List the three types of clients that nurses assess and plan health care for.

11. List the members in the basic family unit.

12. List the healthy indicators from *Healthy People 2010* that will be achieved through family behaviors.

13. Name the types of households the way the government groups them.

14. List five reasons for single parenthood.

15. List four stresses of single parenthood.

16. List the organ systems that the biologic system can be subdivided into.

17. List the main functions of the family.

18. List the purposes of the family assessment that is used to determine the level of family functioning.

19. List areas of vulnerability of family units to health problems.

20. List four diseases that are preventable or can be minimized or delayed through lifestyle modifications.

21. List three things that children and adults in healthy, functional families receive.

22. List four areas that are shaped from the family's values and beliefs that are unique to their culture of origin.

23. List five areas where families live.

CASE STUDY

24. The Ahl family relocated to a small midwestern town from Iraq. They are trying to learn the ways and the language of the country. They recently had to take their youngest son to the emergency department for a trauma to his left leg. The nurse caring for him noticed he had other healed marks to the torso and to his legs. She also noted the only person who talked was the father. The mother and the other children sat quietly and did not give eye contact.

    1. What should the nurse be observing for?
    2. What questions should be asked about the injury?
    3. What should the nurse know about the culture differences?
    4. Should this case be considered abuse and be reported to social services?

REVIEW QUESTIONS

25. What is a slow, stressful process of learning the language and customs of a new country?

    a. Accustomation
    b. Acculturation
    c. Assimilation
    d. Accentuation

26. Families with more than two generations living together are called what?

    a. Interracial

    b. Interested

    c. Intergenerational

    d. Integrated

27. Families that consist of unrelated individuals or families who live under one roof are called what?

    a. Cohabitating

    b. Consolidated

    c. Conspirators

    d. Controllers

28. What theorist introduced the systems theory as a universal theory that could be applied to many fields of study especially for nurses to understand systems in families and communities?

    a. Skinner

    b. Piaget

    c. Gilligan

    d. von Bertalanffy

29. Name the mechanism by which some of the output of a system is returned to the system as input.

    a. Feedback

    b. Throughput

    c. Negative feedback

    d. Positive feedback

30. Nurses care for clients but also provide care for the family members since they impact the health, values, and productivity of individual family members. What is this type of nursing called?

    a. Family unit nursing

    b. Functional family nursing

    c. Family-centered nursing

    d. Family structured nursing

31. What happens when families of a particular culture cluster to form mutual support systems to preserve their heritage?

    a. They become isolated from other cultures.

    b. This practice may isolate them from the larger society.

    c. They form large communities of a given culture.

    d. Their language skills will be weak.

CHAPTER 11 / Promoting Health in the Family

32. What roles do the parents in a traditional home have?

    a. Both parents work outside the home.

    b. The children attend boarding school.

    c. Women clean and cook, and men take out the garbage and do the yard work.

    d. The mother often assumes the nurturing role and the father provides the necessary economic resources.

33. "Two adults who have chosen to share one another's lives in an intimate and committed relationship of mutual caring" is the definition of which of the following?

    a. Marriage

    b. Lesbian relationship

    c. Domestic partnership

    d. Heterosexual relationship

34. How did Dorothy Johnson describe the human system?

    a. As a holistic view

    b. In terms of behaviors

    c. In subsystems

    d. As psychologic subsystems of attachment

35. What does the structural–functional theory focus on?

    a. Family structure and function

    b. The action of the family

    c. Membership of the family

    d. Relationships among family members

CHAPTER 12

CARING

KEY TERM REVIEW

Match each term with its appropriate definition.

1. _____ Aesthetic knowing
2. _____ Caring
3. _____ Caring practice
4. _____ Empirical knowing
5. _____ Ethical knowing
6. _____ Personal knowing
7. _____ Reflection

a. The promotion of wholeness and integrity in the personal encounter, achieves engagement rather than detachment, and denies the manipulative or impersonal approach

b. Ranges from factual, observable phenomena (e.g., anatomy, physiology, chemistry) to theoretical analysis (e.g., developmental theory, adaptation theory)

c. Thinking from a clinical point of view, analyzing why one acted in a certain way, and assessing the results of one's actions

d. The art of nursing expressed by the individual nurse through his or her creativity and style in meeting the needs of clients

e. People, relationships, and things that matter

f. Connection, mutual recognition, and involvement

g. A focus on matters of obligation or what ought to be done, and goes beyond simply following the ethical code of discipline

EXPLORE mynursingkit
www.mynursingkit.com

MyNursingKit is your one stop for online chapter review materials and resources. Prepare for success with additional NCLEX®-style practice questions, interactive assignments and activities, web links, animations and videos, and more! Register your access code from the front of your textbook at www.mynursingkit.com

Look for these resources:
- NCLEX® Review
- Case Studies
- Videos and Animations

CHAPTER 12 / Caring

KEY TOPIC REVIEW

8. List the eight major ingredients of the caring process.

9. List the five different definitions of caring as identified by Morse, Solberg, Neander, Battorff, and Johnson.

10. List the 6 Cs of caring.

11. List the four important modes in the aesthetic pattern of knowing.

12. List the three areas that caring encounters are influenced by.

13. List concepts that humans use to develop their caring abilities.

14. List the end products of caring as the moral ideal of nursing.

15. List four concepts of how human caring is related to intersubjective human responses.

16. List the four types of knowledge that are integrated to guide nursing practice.

17. List the goals of nursing.

18. List four ways the nurse assesses a client's pain.

19. List eight things included in enabling.

CASE STUDY

20. As part of the admission process for nursing schools, students are interviewed by the administrator and one of the questions is "Why do you want to be a nurse?" The pat answer is always that they enjoy caring for others. Nursing continues to evolve and change, especially with advanced technology. We often seem to be caring for machines rather than clients, but nurses have to remember that the client always comes first. The nursing profession provides autonomy and areas for growth through continued education and experience. Nurses are employed from staff nurses to educators and can continue to grow personally and professionally.

    1. What happens when you no longer feel like caring for others?
    2. How do nurses continue to give of themselves day in and day out?
    3. How do schools know which students will make good nurses?
    4. What is your goal for the next 10 years?

REVIEW QUESTIONS

21. Which theorist proposed that caring is the essence of nursing, and the distinct, dominant, central, and unifying focus of nursing?

    a. Leininger
    b. Wrubel
    c. Swanson
    d. Watson

22. What theorist wrote the theory of culture care diversity and universality, which is based on the assumption that nurses must understand different cultures in order to function effectively?

    a. Watson

    b. Wrubel

    c. Swanson

    d. Leininger

23. What noted philosopher has proposed that to care for another person is to help him grow and actualize himself?

    a. Ray

    b. Mayeroff

    c. Swanson

    d. Watson

24. Whose theory suggests that caring in nursing is contextual and is influenced by the organizational structure?

    a. Watson

    b. Swanson

    c. Leininger

    d. Ray

25. What did Watson call the process through which the nurse enters into the experience of the client, and the client can enter into the nurse's experience?

    a. Commitment to caring

    b. Common humanity

    c. Possibility of giving

    d. Transpersonal human caring

26. What is Swanson's category that provides a description of nursing presence?

    a. Being with

    b. Emotionally present

    c. Promise of availability

    d. Not emotionally present

27. What medical association wrote that "the nurse has a responsibility to model healthy behaviors"?

    a. American Nurses Association

    b. National League of Nursing

    c. Joint Commission on Accreditation of Healthcare Organizations

    d. American Holistic Nurses Association

28. What must student nurses do in order to develop themselves as caring practitioners?

    a. Nursing schools need to teach them how to care.

    b. They should come from a caring family.

    c. Practice must be personal and meaningful.

    d. They must care about themselves first.

29. Nursing students will learn more and be better prepared as they go through their educational process with the help of which of the following?

    a. Family member

    b. Mentor

    c. Fellow student

    d. Textbook

CHAPTER 13

COMMUNICATION

KEY TERM REVIEW

Match each term with its appropriate definition.

1. _____ Attentive
2. _____ Congruent conversation
3. _____ Decode
4. _____ Elderspeak
5. _____ Empathy
6. _____ Encoding
7. _____ Feedback
8. _____ Group
9. _____ Group dynamics
10. _____ Helping relationship
11. _____ Personal space
12. _____ Process recording
13. _____ Proxemics
14. _____ Territoriality
15. _____ Therapeutic communication

a. An intellectual process that involves correctly understanding another person's emotional state and point of view and an emotional response experienced by the helper

b. Communication that takes place between members of any group

c. Promoting understanding to help establish a constructive relationship between the nurse and the client

d. The distance people prefer in interaction with others

e. The response that a receiver returns to the sender; can be verbal, nonverbal, or both

f. To listen actively using all the senses; a highly developed skill, learned with practice

g. A concept of the space and things that any individual considers belonging to the self

h. A nurse–client relationship that is referred to by some as an interpersonal relationship, by others as a therapeutic relationship

i. The verbal and nonverbal aspects of the message match

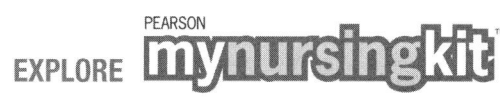

EXPLORE **mynursingkit**

www.mynursingkit.com

MyNursingKit is your one stop for online chapter review materials and resources. Prepare for success with additional NCLEX®-style practice questions, interactive assignments and activities, web links, animations and videos, and more! Register your access code from the front of your textbook at www.mynursingkit.com

Look for these resources:
- NCLEX® Review
- Case Studies
- Videos and Animations

58 CHAPTER 13 / Communication

j. The selection of specific signs or symbols (codes) to transmit the message, such as which language and words to use, how to arrange the words, and what gestures to use

k. The study of distance between people in their interactions

l. Relate the message perceived to the receiver's storehouse of knowledge and experience to sort the meaning of the message

m. A speech style similar to baby talk that gives the message of dependence and incompetence to older adults

n. Two or more people who have shared needs and goals, who take each other into account for their actions, and who are held together and set apart from others by virtue of their interaction

o. A verbatim (word-for-word) account of a conversation

KEY TOPIC REVIEW

16. List the two main purposes for communication.

17. List the five areas that help nurses work more effectively through communication skills.

18. Name the four things that face-to-face communication involves.

19. What are the two ways communication is generally carried out?

20. List four things incorporated in body language.

21. List five feelings that can be expressed by facial expressions.

22. List the keys to a helping relationship.

23. List eight areas that can affect the development of the nurse–client relationship.

24. List four things that should happen between a nurse and a client after the introductory phase of a working relationship.

25. Name the two major stages during the working phase of a relationship.

26. In nursing, communication is a dynamic process. List three things it is used for.

27. List eight terms nurses need to consider when choosing words to say or write.

CASE STUDY

28. Charlie is a 62-year-old male who has displayed signs of dementia for the last six months. He was admitted to the hospital when his wife had a problem getting him out of bed. He was incontinent and did not seem to understand verbal commands. When he does respond, he is very defiant. He recently retired. Before this incident, no physical or medical problems were noted. He is of average height and weight and does not take any prescribed medications. The nurse assigned to the client is struggling to communicate with him. Charlie's wife has no medical background and fears his condition will get worse and that she will not be able to care for him.

    1. What would be a nursing diagnosis needed to address the communication problem?

    2. What is a possible medical diagnosis for his condition?

3. What would be some useful things to teach the wife to better care for her husband?

4. How should the nurse communicate with him so that he will understand and comply?

REVIEW QUESTIONS

29. A message transmitted to another is prepared in a way that will reach the receiver so that he or she understands it. It requires evaluating the language, arranging the words, choosing a tone, and selecting the appropriate gestures. What is this called?

    a. Enhancing

    b. Interpreting

    c. Encoding

    d. Communicating

30. What is the most common form of electronic communication where an individual can send a message, by computer, to another person or group of people?

    a. Snail mail

    b. E-mail

    c. Fax

    d. Webcast

31. Communication has many processes that can enhance or mislead what the sender is trying to say. A message must be sent and received with the meaning intact. What part of the process conveys an attitude of caring and interest?

    a. Listening

    b. Therapeutic communication

    c. Feedback

    d. Attentive listening

32. What style of communication is often perceived as a personal attack by the other person and can humiliate, dominate, control, or embarrass the other person?

    a. Assertive

    b. Aggressive

    c. Attentive

    d. Assistive

33. The nurse is admitting a client to the unit after he suffered a minor stroke. He has physical deficits to his right side and problems responding. What strategy should the nurse use to ensure that the client understands?

    a. Determine if the client can hear.

    b. Determine if the client can use blinking to answer yes or no questions.

    c. Use only open-ended questions when talking to the client.

    d. Have the client's spouse relay information to the client.

34. Nurses need to communicate not only with clients but also with physicians and other staff members. How do they differ in their communication styles?

    a. Nurses are narrative and descriptive and strive for consensus whereas physicians focus on a problem and rule out alternatives.

    b. Nurses follow a set of criteria to evaluate and physicians diagnose and write orders.

    c. Nurses listen and doctors tell them what to do.

    d. Nurses speak in laymen terms whereas physicians speak in medical terms.

35. Nurses provide the client evaluation and a report on the client's progress during an end-of-shift report. These reports are often taped. One way you can ensure that your communication style is effective is to:

    a. ask the other nurse if he or she understood your report.

    b. do nothing. Giving the facts about your clients should be enough.

    c. play back the tape and listen to see if what you wanted to convey was on the tape.

    d. wait for the yearly peer review and see what others think of you.

36. What type of questions should a nurse ask that will assist in obtaining accurate information about the effectiveness of communication?

    a. Closed

    b. Open-ended

    c. Nonverbal

    d. Verbal

37. Nurses need to understand that the layperson does not have a medical background and the terms used should be common ones that everyone would understand. What is another important aspect to ensure clarity in communication?

    a. Listen carefully.

    b. Use eye contact.

    c. Communicate in a well-lit room.

    d. Speak slowly and enunciate carefully.

38. Nurses should be aware of changes in a client by watching for a change in dressing, grooming, and general appearance. How can this be validated?

    a. Through observation

    b. Through discussions with the family

    c. By asking the client

    d. By reading the client's chart

39. When a nurse uses the process of active listening, it involves paying attention to the total message and requires energy and concentration. What form of communication needs to be used to convey the correct message?

    a. Verbal and nonverbal

    b. Congruent

    c. Open-ended

    d. Closed

40. What enables the client to express thoughts and feelings openly with the nurse?

    a. Trust
    b. Risk
    c. Attitude
    d. Interest

41. What is it called when the nurse is able to show an understanding of the client's feelings and the behavior and experience underlying these feelings?

    a. Genuine
    b. Empathy
    c. Compatible
    d. Maturation

CHAPTER 14

TEACHING

KEY TERM REVIEW

Match each term with its appropriate definition.

1. _____ Adherence
2. _____ Affective domain
3. _____ Andragogy
4. _____ Behavioral theory
5. _____ Cognitive domain
6. _____ Cognitive theory
7. _____ Compliance
8. _____ Geragogy
9. _____ Health literacy
10. _____ Humanism
11. _____ Imitation
12. _____ Learning
13. _____ Learning need
14. _____ Modeling
15. _____ Motivation
16. _____ Pedagogy
17. _____ Psychomotor domain
18. _____ Readiness
19. _____ Teaching

a. An individual's desire to learn and to act on the learning

b. A system of activities intended to produce learning

c. The process involved in stimulating or helping older adults to learn

d. The desire to learn

e. The focus on the feelings and attitudes of learners, on the importance of the individual in identifying learning needs and in taking responsibility for them, and on the self-motivation of the learners to work toward self-reliance and independence

f. The art and science of teaching adults

g. A commitment or attachment to a regimen

h. The process by which a person learns by observing the behavior of others

i. The "skill" domain, which includes motor skills such as giving injections

j. The "feeling" domain, which is divided into categories that specify the degree of a person's depth of emotional response to tasks

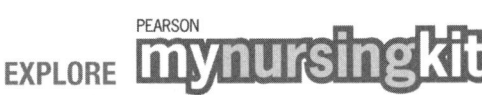

EXPLORE mynursingkit

www.mynursingkit.com

MyNursingKit is your one stop for online chapter review materials and resources. Prepare for success with additional NCLEX®-style practice questions, interactive assignments and activities, web links, animations and videos, and more! Register your access code from the front of your textbook at www.mynursingkit.com

Look for these resources:
- NCLEX® Review
- Case Studies
- Videos and Animations

k. The "thinking" domain, which includes six intellectual abilities and thinking processes, beginning with knowing, comprehending, applying with analysis, synthesis, and evaluation

l. The ability to read, understand, and act on health information, including such tasks as comprehending

m. The process by which individuals copy or reproduce what they have observed

n. The discipline concerned with helping children learn

o. Identifying what is to be taught; immediately identifying and rewarding correct responses

p. A desire or a requirement to know something that is presently unknown to the learner

q. Recognizing the development level of the learner, and acknowledging the learner's motivation and environment

r. A change in human disposition or capability that persists and cannot be solely accounted for by growth

s. The demonstration of behaviors or cues that reflect the learner's motivation to learn at a specific time

KEY TOPIC REVIEW

20. List the areas that the provider must consider when a client is educated by nurses.

21. List three components of client care.

22. What does each participant contribute in the teaching–learning process?

23. List four andragogic concepts about adult learners that should be used as a guide for client teaching.

24. List three main theoretical constructs.

25. List Piaget's five major phases of cognitive development.

26. List Lewin's four different types of changes.

27. List Lewin's three basic stages in his theory of change.

28. Identify Bloom's three domains or areas of learning.

29. List three ways of providing positive feedback.

30. List barriers to learning.

31. List the six intellectual abilities and thinking processes related to the cognitive domain, the "thinking" domain.

CHAPTER 14 / Teaching

CASE STUDY

32. John was diagnosed with colon cancer and underwent a bowel resection with a colostomy. After the procedure the enterostomal nurse worked with him to explain how to care for the colostomy. He did not look at or touch the colostomy and told the nurse to teach his wife how to do it because he would not take care of it and was embarrassed by having it. He felt he could not lead a normal life and would rather not live if he had to "wear that bag."

   1. How can the nurse teach the client that he can lead a normal life?
   2. What will be the best way to teach him colostomy care?
   3. Should the nurse ask the physician for a consult for social services?
   4. Is it OK that the wife cares for the colostomy to make it easier to prepare the client for discharge?

REVIEW QUESTIONS

33. What agency expanded its standards to include that client education by nurses show evidence that patients and their significant others understand what they have been taught?

    a. ANA

    b. OBRA

    c. AMA

    d. JCAHO

34. What behavior theorist's major contribution that applied to teaching was that learning should be based on the learner's behavior?

    a. Skinner

    b. Pavlov

    c. Thorndike

    d. Bandura

35. What behavior theorist claimed that most learning comes from observational learning and instruction rather than trial-and-error behavior?

    a. Bandura

    b. Skinner

    c. Pavlov

    d. Thorndike

36. When nurses assess their clients' readiness to learn, they must also ask the clients how they learn the best. This helps nurses to determine which of the following for the client?

    a. Support system

    b. Learning style

    c. Teaching style

    d. Lifestyle

37. A problem that continues to exist is illiteracy. We continue to have a huge population who do not have the ability to read and comprehend. They may also not be able to understand instructions to provide care for themselves. Nurses should be aware if any of these issues exist. What is a consequence that could result from these issues?

    a. Clients have better than average health outcomes.

    b. Clients have lower rates of hospitalization.

    c. Clients do not seek information on their health issues.

    d. Clients take the correct medications.

38. When clients have a problem with reading and understanding directions, why do they not just admit to the nurse that they cannot read?

    a. They do not feel it is a problem.

    b. Clients may be too embarrassed to admit they cannot read.

    c. They know someone else can read for them.

    d. The nurse would not believe them.

39. When a client has a reading problem, which NANDA diagnosis should be identified?

    a. *Deficient Knowledge* related to minimal reading skills

    b. *Health-Seeking Behavior*

    c. *Noncompliance*

    d. *Anxiety* related to deficient knowledge

40. A client is ready to be discharged, and all the teaching was completed with the client and spouse. What statement by the client will ensure that the family is prepared with the knowledge to provide the care needed?

    a. I can go home and resume my activities as before.

    b. I should take it easy and reread the instructions when I get home so that I can follow them to improve my health.

    c. The limitations refer to other clients but not to me.

    d. I will have my spouse worry about what I should do and what I should eat.

41. What term(s) did Bastable use to refer to the "ability to maintain health-promoting regimens, which are determined largely by a health care provider"?

    a. Behavioristic

    b. Developmental task

    c. Compliance and adherence

    d. Dependence to independence

42. Which theorist should nurses include in their teaching plan, such as teaching a client how to self-administer insulin is in the psychomotor domain?

    a. Grey's

    b. Skinner's

    c. Bloom's

    d. Maslow's

43. What is it called when a nursing student recognizes a need and believes the need will be met through learning?

    a. Perception

    b. Ambition

    c. Motivation

    d. Application

44. A teaching plan is a written plan consisting of learning outcomes. When the plan is ineffective, what should the nurse do to ensure the client learns the goals needed to promote health?

    a. Revise the plan.

    b. Reeducate the client.

    c. Don't worry about it.

    d. Have someone else do the teaching.

CHAPTER 15

LEADING, MANAGING, AND DELEGATING

KEY TERM REVIEW

Match each term with its appropriate definition.

1. _____ Autocratic leader
2. _____ Bureaucratic leader
3. _____ Change agents
4. _____ Charismatic leader
5. _____ Democratic leader
6. _____ First-level manager
7. _____ Formal leader
8. _____ Informal leader
9. _____ Laissez-faire
10. _____ Leader
11. _____ Leadership style
12. _____ Manager
13. _____ Mentors
14. _____ Middle-level manager
15. _____ Power
16. _____ Preceptor
17. _____ Risk management
18. _____ Role model
19. _____ Shared governance
20. _____ Shared leadership

a. Individuals who initiate, motivate, and implement change

b. Traits, behaviors, motivations, and choices used by individuals to effectively influence others

c. A mental image of a possible and desirable future state

d. An appointed leader selected by an organization and given official authority to make decisions and act

e. Organizational executives responsible for establishing goals and developing strategic plans

f. Influences others to work together to accomplish a goal

g. Recognizing that a professional workforce is made up of many leaders

h. One who does not trust self or others to make decisions, and instead relies on the organization's rules, policies, and procedures to direct the group's work effort

i. Organizational executives responsible for establishing goals and developing strategies

j. Those who give their time, energy, and material support to teach, guide, assist, counsel, and inspire a younger nurse

EXPLORE mynursingkit

www.mynursingkit.com

MyNursingKit is your one stop for online chapter review materials and resources. Prepare for success with additional NCLEX®-style practice questions, interactive assignments and activities, web links, animations and videos, and more! Register your access code from the front of your textbook at www.mynursingkit.com

Look for these resources:
- NCLEX® Review
- Case Studies
- Videos and Animations

21. _____ Situational leader
22. _____ Top-level manager
23. _____ Transactional leader
24. _____ Transformational leader
25. _____ Upper-level management
26. _____ Vision

k. An effective leader showing sensitivity and demonstrating caring toward co-workers and clients

l. Responsibility for managing the work of nonmanagerial personnel and the day-to-day activities of a specific work group or groups

m. Someone who flexes task and relationship behaviors, considers the staff members' abilities, knows the nature of the task to be done, and is sensitive to the context or environment in which the task takes place

n. A leader who recognizes the group's need for autonomy and self-regulation

o. A method that aims to distribute decision making among a group of people

p. An official not officially appointed to direct the activities of others, but because of seniority, age, or special abilities, is recognized by the group as its leader

q. An employee of an organization who is given authority, power, and responsibility for planning, organizing, coordinating, and directing the work of others, and for establishing and evaluating standards

r. A leader who encourages group discussion and decision making

s. A system in place to reduce danger to clients and staff

t. Supervision of a number of first-level managers and responsibility for the activities in the departments they supervise

u. A leader who makes decisions for the group

v. One who has a relationship with followers based on an exchange for some resource valued by the follower

w. A rare individual who is characterized by an emotional relationship between the leader and the group members

x. One who fosters creativity, risk taking, commitment, and collaboration by empowering the group to share in the organization's vision

y. The relationship in which the experienced nurse assists the "new" nurse in improving clinical nursing skills and judgment

z. A person's ability to control the environment

KEY TOPIC REVIEW

27. List aspects that are consistent components of the nurse's role.

28. List six attributes of a leader.

29. List the purposes of nursing leadership.

30. List specific traits and abilities leaders often possess.

31. List four leadership styles.

32. List four responsibilities of a nurse manager.

33. List four theories about the situational leader.

CHAPTER 15 / Leading, Managing, and Delegating 69

34. List five descriptive factors that make a leader effective.

35. List five things that are needed to be a good leader.

36. List the eight functions that help to achieve the broad goal of quality client care.

37. List five steps of risk management.

38. List eight things that are needed to be effective managers.

CASE STUDY

39. A new graduate nurse arrived on the pediatric unit for her first day on the job. She was on the unit during her clinical rotation and had decided to apply for a position. She was offered a third-shift position with orientation for two weeks on the day shift. She was very nervous about caring for children because their needs are different from adults and medications are calculated by age and weight. She will be working with a senior nurse who has worked on the unit for seven years. The first thing she needed to do was to meet with the nurse manager and receive an orientation packet that will guide her through the skills she will need to be signed off on. Her first impression of the manager was that she listened to the staff nurses and let them do whatever they thought was correct.

    1. What is the person called who will work with the new graduate nurse?
    2. What style of leadership does the nurse manager practice?
    3. What will the senior nurse provide for the new graduate?
    4. What are some skills that the new graduate will be signed off on to ensure she is a safe practitioner?

REVIEW QUESTIONS

40. What style of leadership is the most effective in the health care system?

    a. Laissez-faire

    b. Autocratic

    c. Democratic

    d. Bureaucratic

41. The five rights of delegation are the right task, under the right circumstances, to the right person, with the right direction and communication, and the right supervision and evaluation. What regulatory agency established the five rights?

    a. ANA

    b. NLN

    c. NCSBN

    d. OBRA

42. Change is an integral aspect of nursing, and nurses are often the individuals who initiate, motivate, and implement change. What is the person called who initiates change?

    a. Change agent

    b. Implementer

    c. Motivator

    d. Changer

© 2011 by Pearson Education, Inc.

CHAPTER 15 / Leading, Managing, and Delegating

43. Whose model for change involves the three stages of unfreezing, moving, and refreezing?

    a. Watson

    b. Lewin

    c. Leininger

    d. Swanson

44. The critical care unit has had the same management and rules for the last 5 years. When the morning staff came on duty, they were greeted with a new manager and new rules and regulations for the operation of the unit. What should the staff do?

    a. They should demand a voice in how the unit should be reorganized.

    b. They should accept the changes without complaints.

    c. They should wait and see what happens with the changes.

    d. They should understand that change is inevitable and does not have to be detrimental to the unit or staff and they should consider what is best for the client.

45. Nurses can delegate tasks to all other staff members if they are qualified and trained in the procedure. Unlicensed personnel can delegate to which of the following?

    a. Nurses

    b. Nurse aides

    c. Housekeeping

    d. No one

46. What is an informal strategy used to gain the cooperation of others without exercising formal authority?

    a. Vision

    b. Role model

    c. Influence

    d. Humanistic

47. Change does not always fit into a person's attitudinal framework, and although change is going to happen it may not always be which of the following?

    a. Accepted

    b. Appreciated

    c. Needed

    d. Wanted

48. What is the difference between a leader and a manager?

    a. Leaders are born; managers are developed.

    b. Leaders are hired; managers are chosen.

    c. Managers are officially appointed; leaders may or may not be appointed.

    d. Leaders manage relationships; managers manage resources.

CHAPTER 16

VITAL SIGNS

KEY TERM REVIEW

Match each term with its appropriate definition.

1. _____ Afebrile
2. _____ Apnea
3. _____ Arrhythmia
4. _____ Basal metabolic
5. _____ Blood pressure
6. _____ Bradycardia
7. _____ Bradypnea
8. _____ Cardiac output
9. _____ Compliance
10. _____ Conduction
11. _____ Convection
12. _____ Diastolic pressure
13. _____ Dysrhythmia
14. _____ Exhalation
15. _____ Expiration
16. _____ Febrile
17. _____ Hypertension
18. _____ Hypotension
19. _____ Hypothermia
20. _____ Inhalation

a. The apical pulse, which is a central pulse, located at the apex of the heart

b. A fast heart rate (e.g., over 100 BPM in an adult)

c. The volume of blood pumped into the arteries by the heart and equals the result of the stroke volume (50) times the heart rate (HR) per minute

d. A blood pressure that is persistently above normal

e. The client who has a fever

f. The dispersion of heat by air currents

g. The intake of air into the lungs

h. The arterial measurement of pressure exerted by the blood as it flows through the arteries

i. The intake of air into the lungs

j. A client who does not have a fever

k. A heart rate of less than 60 BPM in adults

l. A loss that accounts for about 10% of basal heat loss

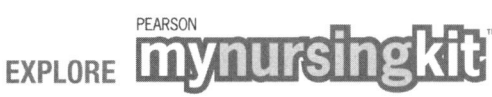

www.mynursingkit.com

MyNursingKit is your one stop for online chapter review materials and resources. Prepare for success with additional NCLEX®-style practice questions, interactive assignments and activities, web links, animations and videos, and more! Register your access code from the front of your textbook at www.mynursingkit.com

Look for these resources:
- NCLEX® Review
- Case Studies
- Videos and Animations

21. _____ Insensible heat loss
22. _____ Inspiration
23. _____ Korotkoff's sounds
24. _____ Orthostatic hypotension
25. _____ Point of maximal impulse
26. _____ Pulse
27. _____ Pulse oximeter
28. _____ Pulse pressure
29. _____ Pyrexia
30. _____ Radiation
31. _____ Respiration
32. _____ Systolic pressure
33. _____ Tachycardia
34. _____ Tachypnea
35. _____ Tidal volume
36. _____ Ventilation

m. A wave of blood created by contraction of the left ventricle of the heart, generally representing the stroke volume output or the amount of blood that enters the arteries with each ventricular contraction

n. A core body temperature below the lower limit of normal

o. Identifying phases in the series of sounds when taking blood pressure with a stethoscope

p. A pulse with an irregular rhythm

q. A blood pressure that falls when the client sits or stands

r. Breathing out or the movement of air in and out of the lungs

s. A body temperature above the usual range or (in lay terms) fever

t. Cessation of breathing

u. A pulse with an irregular rhythm

v. Abnormally slow breathing

w. The transfer of heat from one molecule to a molecule of lower temperature

x. Breathing out, or the movement of air in and out of the lungs

y. The pressure when the ventricles are at rest

z. A blood pressure that is below normal, that is, a systolic reading consistently between 85 and 110 mmHg in an adult whose normal pressure is higher than this

aa. The pressure of the blood as a result of cardiac contraction of the ventricle

bb. During a normal inspiration and expiration when an adult takes in about 500 mL of air

cc. The difference between the diastolic and the systolic pressure

dd. A noninvasive device that estimates a client's arterial blood oxygen saturation (SaO_2) by means of a sensor attached to a finger, toe, nose, earlobe, or forehead (or around the hand or foot of a neonate)

ee. Quick, shallow breaths

ff. Frequency of breathing, recorded as the number of breaths per minute

gg. The transfer of heat from the surface of one object to the surface of another without contact between the two objects, mostly in the form of infrared rays

hh. The rate of energy utilization in the body required to maintain essential activities such as breathing

ii. The ability of the arteries to contract and expand

jj. The movement of air in and out of the lungs

KEY TOPIC REVIEW

37. List the five vital signs.

38. List five factors that affect the body's heat production.

39. List four ways heat is lost from the body.

40. List the three main parts of the system that regulates body temperature.

41. List three physiologic processes to increase the body temperature.

42. List the six factors for the body temperature measurements that deviate from normal.

43. List the reasons why adults over the age of 75 years are at risk of hypothermia (temperatures below 36°C, or 96.8°F).

44. Name the four common types of fevers.

45. List contraindications for the use of rectal temperatures.

46. What eight factors should a nurse consider when assessing a client's pulse?

47. List the nine sites where a pulse may be measured.

CASE STUDY

48. Jane arrived at the doctor's office for her yearly physical exam. She had several issues to discuss with her doctor about health issues that had happened over the past year. She noticed when she got out of bed in the morning that she felt faint and would have to sit back down for a while and then get up slowly. This did not greatly concern her but was annoying. The medical assistant took her back to the exam room and checked her vital signs. The assistant had a problem keeping the blood pressure cuff on her arm. Because of Jane's weight, her arms were large. She asked if a larger cuff should be used but the assistant told her no, that it would work OK. The blood pressure registered 166/92 and the assistant told her that was in a high range.

   1. What was the problem with getting out of bed and feeling faint?

   2. Should the assistant use a larger cuff for obese clients?

   3. Would a larger cuff make a difference in the BP reading?

   4. When Jane discussed the symptoms with the assistant or the physician, what should they have done to check to see if there was a problem?

REVIEW QUESTIONS

49. Where is the center that controls the core temperature of the body?

    a. Cerebellum

    b. Cerebrum

    c. Hypothalamus

    d. Hypothalamic integrator

50. What is the apical pulse referred to as?

    a. Central pulse

    b. Apex

    c. Heartbeat

    d. Point of maximal impulse

51. What is a fast heart rate referred to as?

    a. Bradycardia

    b. Tachypnea

    c. Tachycardia

    d. Orthopnea

52. What are Korotkoff's sounds?

    a. The noise the heart makes when a valve is bad

    b. The noise from a client having pneumonia

    c. Five phases in a series of sounds when taking a BP (they may not always be audible)

    d. The sounds heard when taking a blood pressure

53. Why should a client not be permitted to have a high body temperature for a prolonged period of time?

    a. Heat can damage the parenchyma cells, especially in the brain, and the damage may be irreversible.

    b. The body will change its set point.

    c. The client will become dehydrated.

    d. High fevers can cause seizures.

54. Which set of vital signs should the nurse be most concerned about?

    a. 37.5 88 20 132/78

    b. 38.2 66 14 110/54

    c. 37 74 18 120/82

    d. 39 94 12 80/50

55. What is it called when a client's blood pressure changes dramatically from sitting to standing and can often cause fainting?

    a. Hypotension

    b. Hypertension

    c. Orthostatic

    d. Eupnea

56. What is a noninvasive way to measure a client's oxygen saturation?

    a. Stethoscope

    b. Oximeter

    c. Doppler

    d. Sphygmomanometer

57. Where is the safest site to use for a temperature?

    a. Rectal

    b. Axillary

    c. Tympanic

    d. Oral

58. Wearing wet clothing on a cool day can cause what health problem?

    a. Hyperthermia

    b. Chafing

    c. Hypothermia

    d. Hypotension

59. Where can a blood pressure be performed if the arms are not available?

    a. Brachial

    b. Ankle

    c. Thigh

    d. Wrist

60. Blood pressure can be taken either directly or indirectly. How is it done directly?

    a. Insert a catheter into the brachial, radial, or femoral artery.

    b. Use a Doppler to the apical.

    c. Use a blood pressure cuff on the wrist.

    d. Use a jugular vein to introduce a transducer into the heart.

CHAPTER 17

HEALTH ASSESSMENT

KEY TERM REVIEW

Match each term with its appropriate definition.

1. _____ Adventitious breath sounds
2. _____ Auscultation
3. _____ Blanch test
4. _____ Bruit
5. _____ Cerumen
6. _____ Clubbing
7. _____ Crepitations
8. _____ Dullness
9. _____ Flatness
10. _____ Goniometer
11. _____ Hyperresonance
12. _____ Inspection
13. _____ Intensity
14. _____ Jaundice
15. _____ Lift
16. _____ Normocephalic
17. _____ Otoscope
18. _____ Palpation
19. _____ Percussion
20. _____ Pleximeter

a. A condition in which the angle between the nail and the nail bed is 180 degrees or greater

b. The area an individual can see when looking straight ahead

c. A soft, waxy substance, when dry a grayish-tan color; or sticky in various shades of brown

d. The degree of detail the eye can discern in an image

e. An instrument for measuring joint angles

f. A sound occurring when the atrioventricular (A-V) valves close

g. An extremely dull sound produced by very dense tissue, such as muscle or bone

h. An instrument for examining the interior of the ear, especially the ear drum, consisting essentially of a magnifying lens and a light, and determination of auditory acuity

i. The process of listening to sounds produced in the body

j. Testing of the capillary refill, or peripheral circulation

k. The act of striking the body surface to elicit sounds that can be heard or vibrations that can be felt

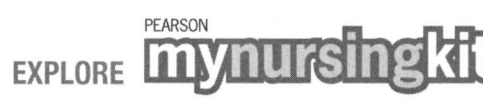

EXPLORE mynursingkit

www.mynursingkit.com

MyNursingKit is your one stop for online chapter review materials and resources. Prepare for success with additional NCLEX®-style practice questions, interactive assignments and activities, web links, animations and videos, and more! Register your access code from the front of your textbook at www.mynursingkit.com

Look for these resources:
- NCLEX® Review
- Case Studies
- Videos and Animations

21. _____ Reflex
22. _____ S$_1$
23. _____ S$_2$
24. _____ Thrill
25. _____ Visual acuity
26. _____ Visual fields

l. Examination of the body by using touch

m. Sounds such as crackles, gurgles, pleural friction rubs, and wheezes

n. The middle finger of the nondominant hand

o. A finding that is not anticipated

p. A heart sound with a high pitch and of short duration described as a "dub"

q. A thud-like sound produced by dense tissue such as the liver, spleen, or heart

r. The visual exam, assessing by using the sense of sight

s. Abnormal breath sounds occurring when air passes through narrowed airways or airways filled with fluid or mucus, or when pleural linings are inflamed

t. A normal head size

u. A vibrating sensation, frequently accompanying a bruit, like the purring of a cat or water running through a hose

v. Automatic response of the body to a stimulus

w. The loudness or softness of a sound

x. A blowing or swishing sound created by turbulence of blood flow due either to a narrowed arterial lumina (a common development in older people) or to a condition such as anemia or hyperthyroidism which elevates cardiac output

y. A yellowish tinge which may first be evident in the sclera of the eyes and then in the mucous membranes and the skin

z. A term referring to a rising along the sternal border with each heartbeat

KEY TOPIC REVIEW

27. List three types of physical examinations.

28. List six purposes for a physical examination.

29. List the four primary techniques used in the physical examination.

30. List ways a nurse can assist a client to relax.

31. List eight terms used to describe skin lesions.

32. List three major considerations to determine the extent of a neurologic exam.

33. List the areas that are assessed in a neurologic exam.

34. What three major areas does the Glasgow Coma Scale assess?

35. Name five reflexes that may be tested during the physical examination.

36. List three functions of the cerebellum.

CHAPTER 17 / Health Assessment

37. List five specific reasons that assessments are performed by nurses.

38. List five types of sound that percussion elicits.

39. List five symptoms of nail fungus.

40. List the four quadrants of the abdomen.

CASE STUDY

41. Tom is having a physical examination by the nurse practitioner. He has not been feeling well for several weeks and has not seen his doctor for two years. He is currently not taking any medications but has started taking some vitamins to help with his lack of energy. He is tired, hungry all the time, thirsty, and frequently urinating. He has lost 7 pounds in the last few months. His vital signs are 37 72 18 126/74. Lungs are clear bilaterally, bowel sounds are active in all quads, and abdomen is soft and nondistended. Height is 5 feet 10 inches, and weight is 245 pounds.

    1. What else should the nurse assess?

    2. What important information should be passed on to the physician?

    3. What questions would the nurse ask to help with the assessment?

    4. What changes will the client need to make to improve his health and what teaching will he need?

REVIEW QUESTIONS

42. What is the medical term for listening?

    a. Palpation

    b. Auscultation

    c. Inspection

    d. Assessment

43. What test is used to detect cancer of the cervix?

    a. Cytology

    b. Vaginal speculum

    c. Pap smear

    d. Papanicolaou test

44. A nurse was teaching her female client to do a self breast exam. Where should she check when checking the tail of Spence?

    a. Below the areola

    b. Under the breast

    c. Axilla area

    d. Above the nipple

45. When assessing skin color, it is best to assess under what kind of light?

    a. Fluorescent light

    b. Natural light

    c. Black light

    d. 100-watt light bulbs

46. To detect jaundice in an African American client, what should you check?

    a. Palms of the hands

    b. Bottoms of feet

    c. Ears

    d. Eyes

47. How can you determine if a client is dehydrated?

    a. Check the amount of fluids taken in.

    b. Check the specific gravity of urine.

    c. Lift and pinch the skin on an extremity.

    d. Assess mucous membranes.

48. In assessing clients, what are white spots on the nails a sign of?

    a. Too much calcium

    b. Iron deficiency

    c. Too much polish

    d. Zinc deficiency

49. When assessing memory, the average person can repeat a series of:

    a. 8–10 digits in sequence and 1–3 digits in reverse

    b. 5–6 digits in sequence and 4–6 digits in reverse

    c. 4–6 digits in sequence and 5–6 digits in reverse

    d. 9–12 digits in sequence and 8–10 digits in reverse

50. In assessing the thyroid gland, the nurse must:

    a. palpate the exterior neck.

    b. stand in front and visualize the neck.

    c. stand to the right of the client and observe as the client swallows water.

    d. auscultate over the thyroid area.

51. What does PERRLA stand for?

    a. Pupils equal round and react to light and accommodation

    b. Periphery evaluation rigid and round left only

    c. Pupils equal reactive to left anteriorly

    d. Pupils equal red laterally assessed

52. Nurses need to have a good understanding of the equipment used to assess clients. One of the most often used items is the stethoscope. How should it be placed in the ears to get the best sound?

    a. The earpieces should be facing forward.

    b. The earpieces should face toward the back.

    c. The earpieces should be comfortable.

    d. The earpieces should be tight.

53. Nurses use all their senses to perform an assessment on a client. The nurse uses the sense of smell to detect unusual odors, especially in the skinfolds or in the axilla. What are these pungent odors from foul-smelling perspiration called?

    a. Poor hygiene

    b. Lack of deodorant

    c. Bromhidrosis

    d. Hyperhidrosis

54. What is the medical term used for an in-grown nail?

    a. Onychomycosis

    b. Hyperhidrosis

    c. Paronychia

    d. Cyanosis

55. What causes dental cavities and periodontal disease?

    a. Poor oral hygiene

    b. Not brushing the teeth

    c. Not scraping the tongue

    d. Plaque and tartar buildup

56. What deformity can rickets cause to the chest?

    a. Kyphosis

    b. Osteoporosis

    c. Pigeon chest

    d. Funnel chest

57. What is the sound of bone grating on bone called?

    a. Crepitation

    b. Grinding

    c. Grating

    d. Tremor

CHAPTER 18

PAIN MANAGEMENT

KEY TERM REVIEW

Match each term with its appropriate definition.

1. _____ Acute pain
2. _____ Allodynia
3. _____ Agonist-analgesia
4. _____ Agonist-antagonist
5. _____ Chronic pain
6. _____ Coanalgesic
7. _____ Dysesthesia
8. _____ Effleurage
9. _____ Equianalgesia
10. _____ Hyperalgesia
11. _____ Nerve block
12. _____ Neurectomy
13. _____ Neuropathic pain
14. _____ Nociception
15. _____ Nonsteroidal anti-inflammatory drugs (NSAIDs)
16. _____ Pain
17. _____ Pain management
18. _____ Pain tolerance

a. Pain that is prolonged, usually recurring or persisting over six months or longer, or interferes with functioning

b. The physiologic processes related to pain perception

c. The interruption of the anterior or posterior nerve root between the ganglion and the cord

d. A term used to denote heightened response to painful stimuli

e. Pain that is directly related to tissue injury and resolves when tissue heals

f. Pain that originates in the skin, muscles, bone, or connective tissue

g. The maximum amount of painful stimuli a person is willing to withstand without seeking avoidance of the pain

h. An "unpleasant sensory and emotional experience associated with actual or potential tissue damage, or described in terms of such damage"

i. Pain arising from organs often presenting as arising from a different area

j. The alleviation of pain or a reduction of pain to a level of comfort that is acceptable to the client

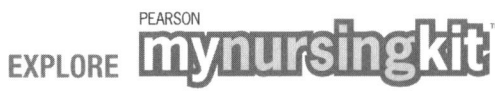

EXPLORE mynursingkit

www.mynursingkit.com

MyNursingKit is your one stop for online chapter review materials and resources. Prepare for success with additional NCLEX®-style practice questions, interactive assignments and activities, web links, animations and videos, and more! Register your access code from the front of your textbook at www.mynursingkit.com

Look for these resources:
- NCLEX® Review
- Case Studies
- Videos and Animations

19. _____ Patient controlled analgesia
20. _____ Placebo
21. _____ Preemptive analgesia
22. _____ Rhizotomy
23. _____ Somatic pain
24. _____ Sympathectomy
25. _____ Transcutaneous electrical nerve stimulation
26. _____ Visceral

k. Nonpainful stimuli that produces pain

l. An unpleasant abnormal sensation

m. A chemical interruption of a nerve pathway effected by injecting a local anesthetic into the nerve

n. Pure opioid drugs that produce maximum pain inhibition, such as morphine, oxycodone, and hydromorphone

o. A type of massage consisting of long, slow gliding strokes

p. A method of applying low-voltage electrical stimulation directly over identified pain areas, at an acupressure point along peripheral nerve areas that innervate the pain area, or along the spinal column

q. A drug that can act like opioids and relieve pain when given to a client who has not taken any pure opioids

r. An agent (formerly known as an adjuvant) that is not classified as a pain medication

s. The relative potency of various opioid analgesics compared to a standard dose of parenteral morphine

t. A term used when peripheral or cranial nerves are interrupted to alleviate localized pain, such as pain in the lower leg or foot arising from a vascular occlusion

u. The pathways of the sympathetic division of the autonomic nervous system are severed

v. An interactive method of pain management that permits clients to treat their pain by self-administering doses of analgesics

w. Pain experienced by people who have damaged or malfunctioning nerves

x. Any medication or procedure, including surgery, which produces an effect in a client because of its implicit or explicit intent and not because of its specific physical or chemical properties

y. Drugs such as ibuprofen or aspirin

z. The administration of analgesics prior to an invasive or operative procedure in order to treat pain before it occurs

KEY TOPIC REVIEW

27. List six things that persistent pain can contribute to.

28. What can persistent pain interfere with?

29. List aspects of nursing care for effective pain management.

30. List four terms used to describe pain.

31. List conditions of abnormal pain processing that may signal the development of neuropathic processes.

32. List four physiologic processes involved in nociception.

33. List factors that can affect a person's perception of, and reaction to, pain.

CHAPTER 18 / Pain Management

34. List four areas that chronic pain affects.

35. List the two major components that pain assessments consist of.

36. List data that should be obtained in a comprehensive pain history.

37. List natural responses to pain.

38. List eight things that the mind–body interventions include.

CASE STUDY

39. Ritchie, a 67-year-old male, was brought into the emergency department by his wife. He was complaining of severe pain to his right foot. The student nurse assigned to him was taking a history and helping him to get undressed. When the client was putting on a hospital gown, he reached down and removed a right leg prosthesis. He had a below-knee amputation several years earlier after a car accident. He has continuously suffered from pain to that limb. The pills he was given for the pain only work for short intervals, and he often comes into the hospital for morphine injections.

   1. What is this type of pain called?
   2. Will medication provide him pain relief?
   3. Is there another way to provide relief for him besides morphine?
   4. This is not a cost-effective approach to providing care. What could be done to provide him with relief without going to the hospital?

REVIEW QUESTIONS

40. When should pain be evaluated?

    a. When the client complains of pain

    b. When the client grimaces

    c. When vital signs are taken

    d. At least once every eight hours

41. Pain felt in one area of the body may be caused from another site. For example, pain to the right shoulder could be from the gallbladder. What is this called?

    a. Chronic pain

    b. Acute pain

    c. Referred pain

    d. Visceral pain

42. What form of pain originates in the skin, muscles, bone, or connective tissue?

    a. Visceral pain

    b. Somatic pain

    c. Referred pain

    d. Acute pain

CHAPTER 18 / Pain Management

43. What type of pain is experienced by people who have damaged or malfunctioning nerves?

    a. Referred pain

    b. Visceral pain

    c. Somatic pain

    d. Neuropathic pain

44. The nurse is attempting to manage a client's chronic pain without success and learns from a review of the literature that evidence suggests this pain results from inadequate treatment during the perioperative period. What type of pain does this client have?

    a. Somatic pain

    b. Referred pain

    c. Neuropathic pain

    d. Chronic pain

45. What is the maximum amount of painful stimuli that a person is willing to withstand without seeking avoidance of the pain or relief?

    a. Pain threshold

    b. Pain acceptance

    c. Pain tolerance

    d. Neuropathic pain

46. A nurse making rounds on a young client noticed he was laughing and having a good time with his visitors. The nurse interrupted and did a set of vitals on the client and asked him to rate his pain. He rated his pain at a 6, which did not seem to match his demeanor. What should the nurse do?

    a. Wait until after the visitors leave and ask him again.

    b. Medicate him because the client should always be believed.

    c. Explain the rating system to the client.

    d. Medicate him with Tylenol and not the Percocet that was ordered.

47. How does the body interpret pain?

    a. It is interpreted as an interaction between the body's analgesia system and the nervous system's transmission.

    b. It is interpreted through chemical mediators.

    c. It follows the nerve endings and becomes inflamed.

    d. It is transmitted to the spine and brain where the signals are modified before they are ultimately understood and detected.

48. How is behavior related to pain as a part of the socialization process?

    a. Cultural background can affect the level of pain that an individual is willing to tolerate.

    b. Tolerance of pain signifies strength and endurance.

    c. Self-infliction of pain is a sign of mourning or grief.

    d. There are significant variations in the expression of pain.

49. How can nurses accurately evaluate pain?

    a. Ask the client.

    b. Use the Wong Baker faces chart.

    c. Use numerical pain intensity scales.

    d. Evaluate the client through activities.

50. Physiologic indicators may vary in infants, so how can pain be determined?

    a. Ask them.

    b. Observe their behavior.

    c. Evaluate the shrillness of their cry.

    d. Observe how they respond to holding.

51. How does having a support system affect pain?

    a. A person without a support network may perceive pain as severe.

    b. The person who has supportive people around may perceive less pain.

    c. A support system helps to alleviate pain.

    d. Friends help to take a person's mind off pain.

52. A client is being discharged after having a shoulder replaced. His pain was controlled with 100 mg of morphine intravenously per day for pain. What oral dose will he need at home that will be equivalent to the dose he was getting?

    a. 300 mg po

    b. 200 mg po

    c. 100 mg po

    d. 400 mg po

53. What are coanalgesics beneficial for?

    a. Reduce the side effects of analgesics

    b. Counteract effects of opioids

    c. Potentiate pain medications

    d. Manage neuropathic pain

54. What is the placebo effect?

    a. Extends the action of the medication

    b. Has an action that reduces pain but may not last long

    c. Can be used for any ailment but results may vary with each individual

    d. Is a perceptible, measurable, and desirable consequence that exceeds the anticipated biologic changes

55. What is the problem with damaging nerves with alcohol, phenol, or radio frequency to eradicate pain?

    a. It doesn't work for everyone.

    b. The nerve endings can grow back and pain will return.

    c. The procedure can be more painful than the pain itself.

    d. They only last for short periods of time.

CHAPTER 19

ASEPSIS

KEY TERM REVIEW

Match each term with its appropriate definition.

1. _____ Active immunity
2. _____ Acute infection
3. _____ Antibodies
4. _____ Antigen
5. _____ Antiseptics
6. _____ Asepsis
7. _____ Autoantigen
8. _____ Bacteria
9. _____ Bloodborne pathogen
10. _____ Cellular immunity
11. _____ Circulating immunity
12. _____ Colonization
13. _____ Disease
14. _____ Disinfectants
15. _____ Exudate
16. _____ Fungi
17. _____ Hyperemia
18. _____ Iatrogenic infections
19. _____ Leukocytosis

a. Proteins that originate in a person's own body

b. A state of infection that can take many forms

c. The most common infection-causing microorganisms

d. Fluid that escaped from the blood vessels, dead phagocytic cells, and dead tissue cells and the products they release

e. A detectable alteration in normal tissue function

f. Consists primarily of nucleic acid and therefore must enter living cells in order to reproduce

g. Agents that destroy pathogens other than spores

h. The freedom from disease-causing microorganisms

i. Microorganisms carried in blood and body fluids that are capable of infecting other persons with serious and difficult to treat viral infections

j. A marked increase in blood supply responsible for characteristic signs of redness and heat

k. A part of the body's plasma proteins

EXPLORE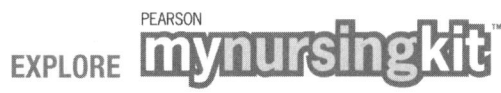

www.mynursingkit.com

MyNursingKit is your one stop for online chapter review materials and resources. Prepare for success with additional NCLEX®-style practice questions, interactive assignments and activities, web links, animations and videos, and more! Register your access code from the front of your textbook at www.mynursingkit.com

Look for these resources:
- NCLEX® Review
- Case Studies
- Videos and Animations

20. _____ Nosocomial infection
21. _____ Parasites
22. _____ Reservoirs
23. _____ Sepsis
24. _____ Sterilization
25. _____ Vector-borne transmission
26. _____ Virus

l. The host produces antibodies in response to natural antigens (e.g., infectious microorganisms) or artificial antigens (e.g., vaccines)

m. Agents that inhibit growth of some microorganisms

n. An infection associated with the delivery of health care services in a health care facility

o. An infection generally having a sudden onset and of short duration

p. A substance that induces a state of sensitivity or immune responsiveness (immunity)

q. Sources of microorganisms

r. The process by which strains of microorganisms become resident flora

s. On exposure to an antigen, the lymphoid tissues release large numbers of activated T cells into the lymph system

t. The defenses that reside ultimately in the B lymphocytes and are mediated by antibodies produced by B cells

u. An animal or flying or crawling insect that serves as an intermediate means of transporting the infectious agent

v. A condition when the bone marrow produces large numbers of leukocytes and releases them into the bloodstream

w. A process that destroys all microorganisms, including spores and viruses

x. Yeasts and molds

y. They live on other living organisms

z. The direct result of diagnostic or therapeutic procedures

KEY TOPIC REVIEW

27. List four areas where microorganisms exist.

28. List the two basic types of asepsis.

29. List four major categories of microorganisms that cause infection in humans.

30. List six ways bacteria are transported.

31. List the most common sites for health care–associated illnesses.

32. List the six links that make up the chain of infection.

33. List five sources of microorganisms.

34. List the three mechanisms of transmission when a microorganism leaves its source or reservoir.

35. List five ways to project droplet spray.

36. List four things that can affect susceptibility to infection.

37. List the five signs of the inflammatory response.

38. List five factors that can influence the development of infection.

39. List four problems caused by prolonged elevation of blood cortisone.

40. List the four strategies set by the campaign to Prevent Antimicrobial Resistance in Healthcare Settings.

41. List three major goals for clients susceptible to infection.

CASE STUDY

42. Sally, an 82-year-old female, was admitted to the hospital with a bowel obstruction and was rushed to the OR for a resection. The surgery went well, but when they tried to extubate her she was not able to breathe on her own. She was placed on a respirator and was eventually taken back to the OR and had a tracheostomy placed for easier access. During her hospital stay she was cultured positive for vancomycin resistant enterococcus (VRE). After several attempts to remove the tracheostomy without success, they decided to transfer her to a skilled care facility for rehabilitation. She has been placed in a private room and has an indwelling catheter. Due to her inability to get out of bed, she is incontinent of feces. She also has an abdominal dressing from the first surgery.

    1. How will the nurses treat the VRE to keep it from spreading?
    2. Why did they place a tracheostomy?
    3. What areas of infection would the nurse be concerned with?
    4. Will the cultures always be positive or is VRE a curable problem?

REVIEW QUESTIONS

43. What organization is known as the major regulatory agency at the international level?

    a. CDC

    b. WHO

    c. OSHA

    d. JCAHO

44. What are infections that are associated with the delivery of health care services in a health care facility?

    a. Nosocomial infections

    b. Health care–associated infections

    c. VRE

    d. MRSA

45. What is the process by which strains of microorganisms become resident flora?

    a. Septicemia

    b. Bacteremia

    c. Colonization

    d. Infections

46. What is the body's first line of defense?

    a. Immune system

    b. Integumentary system

    c. Physiologic barriers

    d. Inflammatory response

47. What is a major underlying disease predisposing clients to infection because of compromised peripheral vascular status and increased serum glucose levels that increase susceptibility?

    a. Diabetes insipidus

    b. Diabetes mellitus

    c. Peripheral vascular disease

    d. Increased cortisone

48. Nurses need to protect clients from infections by teaching them to do which of the following?

    a. Wash hands after contacting a body substance.

    b. Prevent the spread of microorganisms.

    c. Wash hands three times a day.

    d. Maintain hand hygiene when moving from clean to dirty areas.

49. After setting up a sterile field for a dressing change, the nurse was called out of the room for an emergency. When he returns, what should he do about the sterile field and dressing change?

    a. If no one touched it, the nurse can proceed.

    b. The nurse should have the next shift change the dressing.

    c. The nurse should dispose of all open items and set up the sterile field again and change the dressing.

    d. Once the nurse walked away, it is no longer considered sterile.

50. What unusual sign of an infection may be noted in an older adult?

    a. Redness

    b. Swelling

    c. Fever

    d. Disorientation

51. What should nurses do when exposed to a client's blood?

    a. Clean up the area with soap and water.

    b. Report the incident and get tested for hepatitis B and C, and HIV.

    c. Test the client for HIV.

    d. No action is necessary.

52. What is the nurse's goal if infection cannot be prevented?

    a. Prevent the spread of the infection within and between persons, and treat the existing infection.

    b. Provide various antibiotics to impede the growth of bacteria.

    c. Maintain a bacterial free environment.

    d. Keep the client isolated.

53. What do nurses do in implementing infection control procedures?

    a. Keep the hand sanitizers full.

    b. Limit visitors in the client's room.

    c. Use critical thinking and agency policy.

    d. Check the client often for signs of infection.

54. What is the most effective infection control measure?

    a. Sneezing into your shoulder

    b. Showering daily

    c. Taking vitamins

    d. Washing hands

55. What is susceptibility?

    a. Suspecting that germs exist

    b. The degree to which an individual can be affected

    c. The probability that an infection will occur

    d. The presence of a microorganism

56. What does nutrition have to do with infections?

    a. Eating properly keeps you healthy.

    b. Food limits the number of microorganisms.

    c. Adequate nutrition enables tissues to maintain and rebuild themselves.

    d. It helps keep the immune system functioning well.

57. What does a bactericidal do?

    a. Destroys bacteria

    b. Prevents the growth and reproduction of some bacteria

    c. Halts the spread of microorganisms

    d. Is only used in hospitals

CHAPTER 20

DIAGNOSTIC TESTING

KEY TERM REVIEW

Match each term with its appropriate definition.

1. _____ Angiography
2. _____ Anoscopy
3. _____ Ascites
4. _____ Aspiration
5. _____ Colonoscopy
6. _____ Computed tomography
7. _____ Cystoscopy
8. _____ Echocardiogram
9. _____ Electrocardiogram
10. _____ Guaiac test
11. _____ Intravenous pyelography
12. _____ Lumbar puncture
13. _____ Manometer
14. _____ Occult blood
15. _____ Paracentesis
16. _____ Phlebotomist
17. _____ Positron emission tomography
18. _____ Proctoscopy

a. An x-ray procedure that has the unique capability of distinguishing minor differences in the density of tissue

b. A measure of solute concentration in the urine that is a more exact measurement of urine concentration than specific gravity

c. A person from a lab who performs venipuncture, collects the blood specimen for tests ordered by the care provider

d. Radiographic studies used to evaluate the urinary tract where the contrast medium is instilled directly in the kidney via the urethra, bladder, and ureters

e. A test to sense fecal blood content

f. An invasive procedure using radiopaque dye injected into the vessels to be examined

g. The viewing of the rectum

h. A noninvasive test that uses reflected sound waves to visualize the kidneys

i. The removal of excess fluid or air to ease breathing

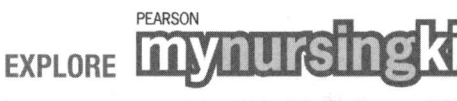

EXPLORE **mynursingkit**

www.mynursingkit.com

MyNursingKit is your one stop for online chapter review materials and resources. Prepare for success with additional NCLEX®-style practice questions, interactive assignments and activities, web links, animations and videos, and more! Register your access code from the front of your textbook at www.mynursingkit.com

Look for these resources:
- NCLEX® Review
- Case Studies
- Videos and Animations

19. _____ Retrograde pyelography
20. _____ Specific gravity
21. _____ Sputum
22. _____ Stress electrocardiography
23. _____ Thoracentesis
24. _____ Trocar
25. _____ Ultrasonography
26. _____ Urine osmolality

j. A noninvasive radiologic study that involves the injection or inhalation of a radioisotope

k. A sharp pointed instrument inside the cannula

l. The use of ultrasound to visualize the structure of the heart

m. Mucous secretion from the lungs, bronchi, and trachea

n. An assessment of a client in response to an increased cardiac workload during exercise

o. The accumulation of a large amount of fluid in the abdominal cavity

p. The viewing of the anal canal

q. The withdrawal of fluid that has abormally collected (e.g., plural cavity, abdominal cavity) or to obtain a specimen (e.g., cerebral spinal fluid)

r. The bladder, ureteral orifices, and urethra are directly visualized using a cystoscope

s. The viewing of the large intestine

t. The drawing of fluid from a site to obtain a specimen or to relieve pressure

u. Radiographic studies used to evaluate the urinary tract where contrast medium is injected intravenously

v. A graphic recording of the heart's electrical activity

w. Hidden blood

x. A glass or plastic tube calibrated in lumbar vertebrae millimeters

y. An indicator of urine concentration or the amount of solutes (metabolic wastes and electrolytes) absent in the urine

z. Cerebrospinal fluid is withdrawn through a needle inserted into the subarachnoid space of the spinal canal between the third and fourth or the fourth and fifth lumbar vertebrae

KEY TOPIC REVIEW

27. List the four most commonly ordered serum tests.

28. List the two blood tests used to evaluate renal function.

29. List three sites where blood gases can be taken.

30. List three foods or items ingested that can show a false-positive result in a Hemoccult test.

31. List five simple urine tests that are done by nurses on the nursing units.

32. List six areas that the MRI is commonly used to visualize.

33. List three reasons why excessive fluid can accumulate in the pleural cavity.

34. List five bones that are commonly used for bone marrow biopsies.

© 2011 by Pearson Education, Inc.

35. List the three phases of diagnostic testing.

36. List five nursing responsibilities associated with specimen collection.

37. List the four structures that can be visualized during a cystoscopy.

38. List four components of a complete blood count (CBC).

CASE STUDY

39. Joan is being admitted for tests to her local hospital for internal bleeding and general malaise. She is scheduled for a 24-hour urine, hematocrit and hemoglobin every 4 hours, Hemoccult of all stool specimens, and a CBC with a chem 6 panel. The nurse's responsibility is to carry out the physician's orders either by performing the tests or by having them done by others.

    1. When should the 24-hour urine test be started?

    2. Why would the physician order hematocrit and hemoglobin every 4 hours?

    3. What would a positive Hemoccult mean?

    4. What is the nurse's responsibility to the client?

REVIEW QUESTIONS

40. What is the most commonly used diagnostic tests that can provide valuable information about the hematologic system and other body systems?

    a. MRI

    b. CAT

    c. Hematology

    d. Urinalysis

41. What is the end product of protein metabolism and is measured as BUN?

    a. Urea

    b. Creatinine

    c. Sodium

    d. Glucose

42. What is a definitive test for hyperglycemia in diabetics that shows results for three to four months prior?

    a. Chemstrip

    b. Glucometer

    c. A_{c1}

    d. Glycosylated hemoglobin

43. What is the test to determine if occult blood is present in feces?

    a. Peroxidase

    b. Hemoccult

    c. Guaiac

    d. Reagent

44. What is a noninvasive radiologic study that involves the injection or inhalation of radioisotopes?

    a. MRI

    b. CAT

    c. PET

    d. LP

45. What abdominal test is carried out to obtain a fluid specimen for laboratory study and to relieve pressure on the abdominal organs due to the presence of excess fluid?

    a. PET

    b. LP

    c. Ascites

    d. Paracentesis

46. A thoracentesis is a procedure to remove the excess fluid or air to ease breathing and can also be used for which of the following?

    a. Perform a biopsy

    b. Place drugs

    c. Culture fluids

    d. Culture and sensitivity

47. What does a high or low WBC count show?

    a. High for bacterial infection, low for viral infection

    b. High for viral infection, low for bacterial infection

    c. Leukocytes that combat infections

    d. Determines the number of circulating cells

48. What is the specific gravity of urine?

    a. 1.000 to 1.035

    b. 1.010 to 1.025

    c. 1.020 to 1.040

    d. 1.015 to 1.020

49. Which phase concentrates on nursing care of the client and the follow-up activities and observations?

    a. Postphase

    b. Intratest

    c. Pretest

    d. Prophase

50. What is a puncture of a vein for collection of a blood specimen called?

    a. Arterial stick

    b. Phlebotomist

    c. Venipuncture

    d. Finger stick

51. What are low RBC counts indicative of?

    a. Polycythemia

    b. Hypervolemia

    c. Hemodilution

    d. Anemia

52. What is one of the most frequently ordered blood tests?

    a. RBC

    b. CBC

    c. WBC

    d. H & H

53. What waste product is produced in relatively constant quantities by the muscles and excreted by the kidneys?

    a. Urea

    b. Bilirubin

    c. Nitrogen

    d. Creatinine

54. Why does a physician order a peak and trough on a drug?

    a. To check for toxic level

    b. To check for a subtherapeutic level

    c. To check for a therapeutic level

    d. To check to see if it is working

CHAPTER 21

SAFETY

KEY TERM REVIEW

Match each term with its appropriate definition.

1. _____ Asphyxiation
2. _____ Bioterrorism
3. _____ Chemical restraint
4. _____ Physical restraint
5. _____ Restraint
6. _____ Safety monitoring device
7. _____ Seizure precautions

a. Safety measures taken to protect clients from injury should they have a seizure

b. Any manual method or physical or mechanical device, material, or equipment attached to the client's body that restricts the client's movement

c. A unit with a position sensitive switch that triggers an audio alarm when the client attempts to get out of the bed or chair

d. A national attack using weapons of viruses, bacteria, and other germs

e. Medications such as neuroleptics, anxiolytics, sedatives, and psychotropic agents used to control socially disruptive behavior

f. The lack of oxygen due to interrupted breathing (suffocation)

g. Any protective device used to limit the physical activity of the client or a part of the body

EXPLORE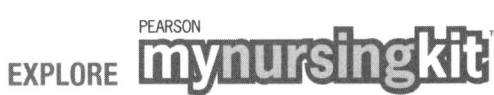

www.mynursingkit.com

MyNursingKit is your one stop for online chapter review materials and resources. Prepare for success with additional NCLEX®-style practice questions, interactive assignments and activities, web links, animations and videos, and more! Register your access code from the front of your textbook at www.mynursingkit.com

Look for these resources:
- NCLEX® Review
- Case Studies
- Videos and Animations

KEY TOPIC REVIEW

8. List six major causes of accidental injury and death.

9. List five lifestyle factors that place people at risk for accidents.

10. List nine factors that affect clients' ability to protect themselves.

11. List five problems in the workplace that can be dangerous.

12. List five things that can create occupational hazards.

13. List four things that contribute to a healthy, hazard-free community.

14. List six areas that a community strives to be free of to remain safe and secure.

15. List six client safety problems.

16. List six factors that increase the risk of human error.

17. List three things involved when assessing clients at risk for accidents and injury.

18. List five perceptual deficits.

19. List six agents of highest concern that can be used for bioterrorism.

20. List three types of facilities that the National Patient Safety Goals are designed for.

21. List seven categories to describe injury more specifically.

22. List important facts regarding suicide of the older adult.

CASE STUDY

23. Frank was diagnosed with dementia and was having problems walking. He was also incontinent and belligerent. He refused to eat at times and was hiding his pills instead of taking them. His family decided they could no longer provide a safe environment in the home and admitted him to a long-term care facility so he could have 24-hour care. He will also receive physical therapy to maintain and improve his physical strength. His second week there he got up during the night and fell, fracturing his left hip and hitting his head, resulting in a concussion.

    1. Was putting him in the facility the best choice?

    2. Are clients with dementia at risk for accidents more often than nondementia clients?

    3. What safety precautions should have been instituted to prevent the fall?

    4. Who is responsible for the fall and the subsequent injuries?

REVIEW QUESTIONS

24. What do more people die from in a given year?

    a. AIDS

    b. Motor vehicle accidents

    c. Breast cancer

    d. Medical errors

25. How does the Institute of Medicine (IOM) define safety?

    a. An injury caused by medical management

    b. Freedom from accidental injury

    c. System flaws set good people up to fail

    d. Adverse events are preventable

26. What tool is available to determine a client's risk for specific kinds of injury, such as falls, or for the general safety of the home and health care setting?

    a. Risk assessment tools

    b. NANDA risk diagnoses

    c. Home hazard appraisal

    d. Community safety risks

27. What are two leading causes of death among teenagers?

    a. Sports accidents and injuries

    b. Suicide and homicide

    c. Motor vehicle accidents

    d. Skin cancer from sun bathing

28. What can nurses do to help prevent our youth from committing suicide?

    a. Educate parents.

    b. Provide educational programs.

    c. Refer to mental health professionals.

    d. Identify behaviors that may indicate potential problems.

29. What is the focus of the National Patient Safety Goals?

    a. Find out if this is the first time the error has happened.

    b. Find out why the error was made.

    c. Find out who made the error.

    d. Find out if the error could have been prevented.

30. Why are older adults' suicide attempts more serious?

    a. They know how to do it.

    b. They are able to purchase guns.

    c. They intend to end their life, not just seek attention.

    d. They have time to plan it.

31. Why are restraints used only as a last measure?

    a. The prn orders are written for the safety of the client.

    b. Clients become more restless and anxious as a result of loss of self-control.

    c. Restraints can be used when the staff is busy.

    d. Families and clients must agree to using restraints.

32. What is the link between nurses' work environment and client safety?

    a. Clients can spread communicable diseases to nursing staff.

    b. Nurses have inconsistent staffing levels and long work hours.

    c. There is a high client to nurse ratio.

    d. Much sicker clients require more nursing time at the bedside.

33. What problem has warranted that nurses be prepared and able to respond appropriately to all types of disasters?

    a. There is always the threat of an intentional attack using weapons of viruses, bacteria, and other germs.

    b. The nursing shortage has created a burden and nurses have to do it all.

    c. More disasters have occurred since September 11, 2001.

    d. A war has lasted longer than eight years.

34. What dangerous health risk threatens children who live in older homes?

    a. Mold in the basements

    b. Lead paint

    c. Open stairways without railings

    d. Black pipes

35. What can help the adolescent experience competition, teamwork, and conflict resolution?

    a. Acquiring a driver's license

    b. Dating

    c. Sports activities

    d. Getting the first job

36. What is domestic violence secondary to?

    a. Mismatched couples

    b. Inability to reconcile differences

    c. Children from previous marriages

    d. Adults who were abused as children

37. What age groups are more prone to falling and having serious injuries?

    a. Infants and toddlers

    b. Toddlers and teens

    c. Infants and older adults

    d. Teens and young adults

38. What should nurses do when they witness a client having a seizure?

    a. Describe their observations before, during, and after.

    b. Protect the client from harm.

    c. Call for help.

    d. Document the incident.

39. What does interrupted breathing lead to?

    a. Seizures

    b. Respiratory and cardiac arrest and death

    c. Poisoning

    d. Suffocation

CHAPTER 22

HYGIENE

KEY TERM REVIEW

Match each term with its appropriate definition.

1. _____ Alopecia
2. _____ Callus
3. _____ Cerumen
4. _____ Cleaning bath
5. _____ Dandruff
6. _____ Dental caries
7. _____ Gingivitis
8. _____ Hygiene
9. _____ Ingrown toenail
10. _____ Pediculosis
11. _____ Periodontal disease
12. _____ Plaque
13. _____ Pyorrhea
14. _____ Scabies
15. _____ Sebum
16. _____ Tartar
17. _____ Therapeutic bath
18. _____ Ticks
19. _____ Xerostomia

a. Loss of teeth due to lack of fluoridated water and preventive dentistry during developmental years

b. A condition that occurs when the supply of saliva is reduced

c. A contagious skin infestation by the itch mite

d. An invisible soft film that adheres to the enamel surface of the teeth

e. The loss of hair

f. An advanced periodontal disease in which the teeth are loose and pus is evident when the gums are pressed

g. Given for physical effects, such as to soothe irritated skin or to treat a specific area

h. A hard, visible deposit of plaque and dead bacteria that forms at the gum line

i. Cavities

j. Small gray-brown parasites that bite into and suck blood, which may transmit diseases to people (e.g., Rocky Mountain spotted fever, Lyme disease, or tularemia)

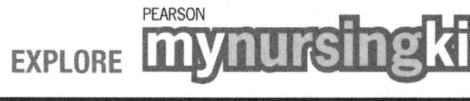

EXPLORE **mynursingkit**

www.mynursingkit.com

MyNursingKit is your one stop for online chapter review materials and resources. Prepare for success with additional NCLEX®-style practice questions, interactive assignments and activities, web links, animations and videos, and more! Register your access code from the front of your textbook at www.mynursingkit.com

Look for these resources:
- NCLEX® Review
- Case Studies
- Videos and Animations

k. A disease characterized by red swollen gingiva, bleeding receding gum lines, and the formation of pockets between the teeth and gums

l. A thickened portion of epidermis or a mass of keratotic material

m. Commonly called earwax

n. Parasites that infest mammals (lice)

o. The growing upward of the nail into the soft tissue around it, most often resulting from improper nail trimming

p. Self-care by which people attend to such functions as bathing, toiletry, and general body grooming

q. Given chiefly for hygiene purposes

r. A diffuse scaling of the scalp

s. An oily substance that (a) softens and lubricates the hair and skin, (b) prevents the hair from becoming brittle, and (c) decreases water loss from the skin when the humidity is low

KEY TOPIC REVIEW

20. List nine areas of care involved in personal hygiene.

21. List the five major functions of the skin.

22. List the chemicals in human sweat.

23. List three areas of assessment of the client's skin and hygienic practices.

24. List eight important considerations when bathing a client.

25. List six ways that the nurse uses to determine and identify clients at risk for foot problems.

26. List six common foot problems.

27. List four organic materials that form plaque on the teeth.

28. List two things that promote dental problems.

29. List four high-risk variables that can contribute to poor oral care.

30. List six things that aggravate a dry mouth.

31. List three effects found in saliva.

32. List five problems with the hair.

33. List three reasons nurses would assess that indicate a client has lice.

34. List the three major functions of brushing hair.

35. List advantages of contacts over eyeglasses.

CASE STUDY

36. Julie was sent to the school nurse because of constantly scratching during class and disrupting the classroom. Her parents had both lost their jobs, and they had lost their home to foreclosure. They have recently been staying in a low-income hotel waiting for housing to open up. The hotel is fairly clean but infestations have been reported in the past.

   1. What type of infestation would make Julie scratch herself?

   2. How should this be treated?

   3. Is there a danger to the other students of catching the infestation?

   4. What has to be done if the infestation came from the hotel?

REVIEW QUESTIONS

37. What is the most common cause of dementia among people age 65 and older?

   a. Organic dementia

   b. Alzheimer's disease

   c. NPH

   d. Brain malfunction

38. What causes a corn (keratosis) to develop?

   a. Pointy shoes

   b. Not wearing socks

   c. Friction and pressure from a shoe

   d. Genetic predisposition

39. How does decay of all the upper teeth and the lower posterior teeth in an infant occur?

   a. Poor oral hygiene

   b. Teeth not being brushed

   c. When an infant is put to bed with a bottle of sugar water, formula, milk, or fruit juice

   d. Teeth appear at birth

40. What is formed when plaque is left on the teeth?

   a. Tartar

   b. Dental caries

   c. Discoloration

   d. Bacteria

41. Why are clients in long-term care settings at higher risk for oral health problems?

   a. They forget to brush because of dementia.

   b. The equipment needed is not readily accessible.

   c. They need to depend on others to provide proper dental care.

   d. They no longer need to care for teeth and usually have dentures.

42. What is a common cause of hearing loss in older adults?

    a. Having the TV too loud

    b. Using headsets from MP3 players

    c. Cerumen buildup

    d. Normal aging process

43. How should nurses wipe loosened secretions from the eyes?

    a. From the inner canthus of the eye to the outer canthus

    b. From the outer canthus of the eye to the inner canthus

    c. From the upper eyelid to the lower eyelid

    d. From the lower eyelid to the upper eyelid

44. What should the nurse do to prevent the eyes from drying out in an unconscious client or one who cannot close the eyes completely?

    a. Rinse eyes gently with tap water.

    b. Keep a moist cloth on the eyes.

    c. Use lubricating eye drops.

    d. Use a chilled eye mask.

45. How do hearing aids work?

    a. Use a volume control to make the sounds around them louder

    b. Block one ear so the other ear hears more sounds

    c. Convert electric energy to sound

    d. Amplify sounds

46. What is the most compact and least visible hearing aid?

    a. Behind-the-ear aid

    b. In-the-ear aid

    c. In-the-canal aid

    d. Body hearing aid

47. Why are hospital beds narrower than a normal bed?

    a. So more beds fit into a room

    b. So nurses can reach both sides of the client

    c. So nurses can reach the client from either side of the bed

    d. So they fit through the doorframe

48. What is the best use for the side rails on a hospital bed?

    a. To keep clients from falling out of bed

    b. To help clients get out of bed

    c. To push the bed from room to room

    d. To provide an arm rest for the client

49. What is a bed cradle used for?

    a. To hold small children

    b. To provide a soothing action for the client

    c. To keep blankets from touching the client

    d. To hold blankets in place

50. Why are bedclothes on a hospital bed mitered?

    a. To keep them from coming out

    b. To keep them looking neat

    c. To secure the bedclothes

    d. To follow hospital protocol

51. When making an occupied bed, what else can the nurse do to use the time wisely?

    a. Assess the client.

    b. Entertain the client.

    c. Change the bed fast and get out.

    d. Mentally make out a grocery list.

CHAPTER 23

MEDICATIONS

KEY TERM REVIEW

Match each term with its appropriate definition.

1. _____ Absorption
2. _____ Agonist
3. _____ Ampule
4. _____ Bevel
5. _____ Biotransformation
6. _____ Buccal
7. _____ Cumulative effect
8. _____ Distribution
9. _____ Drug interaction
10. _____ Drug toxicity
11. _____ Habituation
12. _____ Iatrogenic disease
13. _____ Intradermal
14. _____ Intrathecal
15. _____ Meniscus
16. _____ Parenteral
17. _____ Pharmacodynamics
18. _____ Pharmacokinetics
19. _____ Potentiating effect
20. _____ Stat order

a. Applications that are applied to a circumscribed surface of the body

b. A mild form of psychologic dependence when the individual develops the habit of taking the substance and feels better after taking it

c. An indication a medication is to be given immediately and only once

d. Under the epidermis (into the dermis)

e. A particular type of topical or dermatologic medication delivery system

f. The deleterious effects of a drug on an organism or a tissue

g. Intermittent medications administered through small fluid containers attached below the primary infusion container through the client's IV line

h. The process by which a drug passes into the bloodstream

i. A route for parenteral administration into the tissue just below the skin

j. "Pertaining to the cheek," in which a medication is held in the mouth against the mucous membranes of the cheek until the drug dissolves

21. _____ Subcutaneous
22. _____ Synergistic
23. _____ Topical
24. _____ Transdermal
25. _____ Vial
26. _____ Volume-control infusion set

k. A drug that produces the same type of response as the physiologic or endogenous substance

l. The study of the absorption, distribution, biotransformation, and excretion of a drug

m. The process by which a drug interacts with specific molecules and chemicals normally found in the body

n. A process called detoxification or metabolism by which a drug is converted to a less active form

o. The slanted part at the tip of a needle

p. Intraspinal or into the spinal canal

q. When two different drugs increase the action of one or another drug

r. A small glass bottle in different sizes that can come with a sealed rubber cap

s. An occurrence when the administration of one drug before, at the same time as, or after another drug alters the effect of one or both drugs

t. Disease caused unintentionally by medical therapy

u. The crescent-shaped upper surface of a column of liquid

v. The effect when one or both drugs may be increased

w. A route other than through the alimentary or respiratory tract; that is, by needle

x. The transportation of a drug from its site of absorption to its site of action

y. The increasing response to repeated doses of a drug that occurs when the rate of administration exceeds the rate of metabolic excretion

z. A glass container usually designed to hold a single dose of a drug

KEY TOPIC REVIEW

27. List the four kinds of names for a drug.

28. List six ways drugs are listed and described in the *United States Pharmacopeia (USP)*.

29. List the two pharmacologic effects when a drug binds to its receptor.

30. List two things that nurses need to know about the administration of drugs.

31. List areas where controlled substances are kept.

32. List the information required on an inventory form for controlled substances.

33. List drugs that commonly produce tolerance.

34. List three problems that result from hepatic toxicity.

35. List five over-the-counter drugs that are often overused.

36. List the two types of illicit drugs.

37. List the seven essential parts of a drug order.

38. List six items that should be placed in puncture-proof canisters (generally called sharps containers) that are placed in the client's room.

39. List genetic variations that influence a client's response to a drug.

40. List two things that can affect drug response.

41. List the 10 rights of drug administration.

42. List the major disadvantages of taking oral medications.

43. List three vascular organs where drugs are carried to in the bloodstream.

CASE STUDY

44. Janet, a 42-year-old female, was sent to the hospital for admission after she went to her physician for a nonproductive cough that she had for several weeks. She was running a fever of 102 and had inspiratory wheezing, weakness, general malaise, and chest pain. Vital signs were pulse 92, respirations 22, BP 104/56. Her orders were faxed to the hospital as follows: Tylenol 325mg x2 Q4H prn for temperature >101, codeine elixir 5mL Q4H prn for cough, CXR PA & LAT oxygen 2L nasal cannula, IV DW5 @ 100cc hr, sputum culture.

    1. Are these standardized abbreviations?

    2. What other orders should have been included?

    3. What do you think the diagnoses will be?

    4. What question would be an important part of the history?

REVIEW QUESTIONS

45. If a nurse dispenses a medication written by a physician but the order was unsafe or wrong and the nurse did not question the order, who is responsible?

    a. Nurse

    b. Physician

    c. Pharmacist

    d. Nurse and physician

46. What is it called when a client has an emotional reliance on a drug to maintain a sense of well-being, accompanied by feelings of need or cravings for that drug?

    a. Dependence

    b. Psychologic dependence

    c. Physiologic dependence

    d. Addiction

47. Where would you find lists of drugs and their therapeutic values?

    a. *United States Pharmacopeia*

    b. *National Formulary*

    c. *Nurses' drug guide*

    d. *British Pharmacopoeia*

48. What is a severe allergic reaction that usually occurs immediately after the administration of the drug?

    a. Toxic effect

    b. Cumulative effect

    c. Anaphylactic reaction

    d. Allergic reaction

49. What can delay the dissolution and absorption of some drugs?

    a. Gastric acid

    b. Age of the client

    c. Food in the stomach

    d. Time of day

50. What is the next most rapid route of absorption after intravenous?

    a. Subcutaneous

    b. Intramuscular

    c. Intraosseous

    d. Intrathecal

51. How can genes that control liver metabolism determine how much of a drug should be given?

    a. Slow liver metabolism may achieve an adequate response to a medication.

    b. Rapid metabolizers may require lower doses of a medication to avoid adverse reactions.

    c. Slow metabolizers may require lower doses of a medication to avoid adverse reactions.

    d. Rapid liver metabolism may not achieve an adequate response to a medication.

52. What is ethnopharmacology?

    a. The study of drugs in other countries

    b. The study of the effect of ethnicity on responses to prescribed medication

    c. The study of the genetic ability to produce enzymes that affect drug metabolism

    d. The study of the effect of drugs on animals

53. Where are most metabolites excreted?

    a. Feces

    b. Stomach

    c. Bloodstream

    d. Kidneys

54. Why do nurses need to understand the metric system?

    a. To make things more difficult for nursing students

    b. To confuse their clients with how much medication they are actually getting

    c. To promote a standardized measurement throughout the world

    d. To be able to calculate safe doses for clients since the medications are dispensed in the metric system

55. What can be done to help a client who cannot afford prescriptions or does not have transportation to pick them up?

    a. Contact the client's family to help.

    b. Provide enough medication on discharge.

    c. Contact social services to provide assistance in getting drugs.

    d. Provide referrals to available resources.

56. What is medication reconciliation?

    a. A process to provide the correct drugs to each client

    b. A way to change the medical dispensing system

    c. The process of creating the most accurate list possible of all medications a client is taking

    d. A way to dispense medications more efficiently

57. What is the goal of the Joint Commission's National Patient Safety Goals?

    a. To require a nurse to use at least two client identifiers whenever administering medications

    b. To improve the accuracy of client identification

    c. To use the client's room number as an identifier

    d. To use the wrist band to check the client's ID

58. What is the best way to handle a child when performing a painful procedure?

    a. Tell the child it won't hurt to catch him or her off guard and perform the procedure.

    b. Have the parents hold the child to keep him or her still.

    c. Tell the truth that it will hurt, and cuddle the child afterwards.

    d. Never perform painful procedures in a child's room.

59. What is the unwritten rule when prescribing medications for older adults?

    a. "Start low and go slow."

    b. Less is more.

    c. The fewer medications, the better the client.

    d. Older adults need more medication as they age.

60. What is the danger of parenteral administration of medications?

    a. It is painful for the client.

    b. It is quick acting and is irretrievable once injected.

    c. The nurse could accidentally have a needle stick.

    d. It takes more time than giving a pill.

CHAPTER 24

Skin Integrity and Wound Care

KEY TERM REVIEW

Match each term with its appropriate definition.

1. _____ Approximated
2. _____ Binder
3. _____ Collagen
4. _____ Decubitus ulcers
5. _____ Dehiscence
6. _____ Eschar
7. _____ Evisceration
8. _____ Excoriation
9. _____ Fibrin
10. _____ Granulation tissue
11. _____ Hematoma
12. _____ Hemostasis
13. _____ Ischemia
14. _____ Keloid
15. _____ Maceration
16. _____ Primary intention healing
17. _____ Purulent exudate
18. _____ Pyogenic bacteria
19. _____ Reactive hyperemia
20. _____ Sanguineous exudate

a. A deficiency in the blood supply to the tissue

b. The clear portion of the blood, consisting chiefly of serum derived from blood and the serous membranes of the body

c. A tissue that covers a wound, becoming a translucent red color; is fragile and bleeds easily

d. Wounds left open 3 to 5 days to allow edema or infection to resolve or exudate to drain and then enclosed with sutures, staples, or adhesive skin closures

e. The result of a hypertrophic scar in some individuals, particularly dark-skinned persons, when an abnormal amount of collagen is laid down

f. The process of pus formation

g. A combination of friction and pressure

h. When the tissue surfaces have been closed and there is minimal or no tissue loss

i. The cessation of bleeding

j. Moisture from incontinence which softens tissue and makes the epidermis more easily eroded and susceptible to injury

EXPLORE mynursingkit

www.mynursingkit.com

MyNursingKit is your one stop for online chapter review materials and resources. Prepare for success with additional NCLEX®-style practice questions, interactive assignments and activities, web links, animations and videos, and more! Register your access code from the front of your textbook at www.mynursingkit.com

Look for these resources:
- NCLEX® Review
- Case Studies
- Videos and Animations

21. _____ Secondary intention
22. _____ Serosanguineous
23. _____ Serous exudates
24. _____ Shearing force
25. _____ Suppuration
26. _____ Tertiary intention healing

k. A covering for dressings to prevent the dressing and wound from becoming contaminated

l. A whitish protein substance that adds tensile strength to the wound

m. Clear and blood-tinged drainage commonly seen in surgical incisions

n. Dried plasma and blood covering a wound

o. The area of loss of the superficial layers of the skin, also known as denuded area

p. A localized collection of blood beneath the skin that may appear as a reddish blue swelling (bruise)

q. Pressure sores or bed sores caused by unrelieved pressure on a body area, results in damage to the underlying tissue

r. The protrusion of the internal viscera through an incision

s. Connective tissue

t. A thicker than serous exudate because of the presence of pus, which consists of leukocytes, liquefied dead tissue debris, and living and dead bacteria

u. The tissues have been approximated (closed) and there is minimal or no tissue loss, characterized by the formation of minimal granulation tissue and scarring

v. The bacteria that produces pus

w. A large amount of red blood cells indicating damage to capillaries that is severe enough to allow the escape of red blood cells from plasma

x. When pressure is relieved and the skin takes on a bright red flush

y. A wound, such as a pressure ulcer, that is extensive and involves considerable tissue loss, and in which the edges cannot or should not be approximated

z. The partial or total rupturing of a sutured wound

KEY TOPIC REVIEW

27. List three internal factors that influence skin and skin integrity.

28. List four types of wounds.

29. List eight factors that contribute to the formation of pressure ulcers.

30. List three things that are caused by prolonged inadequate nutrition.

31. List deficiencies that contribute to pressure ulcer formation.

32. List three things that contribute to skin excoriation.

33. List changes in the skin brought on by aging.

34. List six subscales of the Braden Scale for Predicting Pressure Sore Risk.

114 CHAPTER 24 / Skin Integrity and Wound Care

35. List five additional categories from Norton's Pressure Area Risk Assessment Form Scale.

36. List the factors that the rate of healing depends on.

37. List the three phases of wound healing.

38. List the two major processes in the inflammatory phase.

39. List the three major types of exudates.

40. List the three colors of purulent exudates.

41. List characteristics that influence the speed of wound healing.

42. List things clients require in their diet for wound healing.

43. List the signs of shock.

44. List ways sinus tracts are treated when infected.

45. List things the nurse must note when a client has a pressure ulcer.

46. List six nursing interventions for maintaining skin integrity and wound care.

47. List four major areas in which nurses can help clients develop optimal conditions for wound healing.

48. List six body positions clients are placed in.

49. List ways nurses protect red wounds.

50. List the four different ways of debridement.

51. List six reasons for applying dressings.

52. List reasons for different types of dressings used.

CASE STUDY

53. Joshua, a 20-year-old male, arrived in Iraq for his first tour of duty and was assigned to travel with the supply trucks to provide safety for them. Twenty miles from their destination, they hit an IED, and five soldiers were thrown from the burning vehicle. They were triaged and transported to various hospitals. Joshua's injuries included burns over 20% of his upper body along with a fractured femur and numerous lacerations, abrasions, and several open wounds from shrapnel. He was taken to the operating room and had the femur set with screws and all the wounds cleaned and sutured where needed. He will be placed on bed rest with traction and will need to have the burns debrided on a regular basis.

   1. What is the worst injury that he received?

   2. How will he be protected from bed sores while on bed rest?

   3. What will nurses monitor for?

   4. How will they debride the burns?

REVIEW QUESTIONS

54. What is the largest organ in the body?

    a. Liver

    b. Skin

    c. Stomach

    d. Heart

55. What do nurses need to understand about protecting the skin and managing wounds effectively?

    a. Factors affecting skin integrity

    b. The physiology of wound healing

    c. Specific measures that promote optimal skin conditions

    d. The body is healthier when the skin remains intact

56. What happens when blood cannot reach the tissues?

    a. The cells are deprived of oxygen and nutrients.

    b. Waste products of metabolism accumulate in the cells.

    c. The tissue consequently dies.

    d. Breakdowns can occur, especially decubitus ulcers.

57. How can nurses prevent shearing when caring for clients who are bedridden?

    a. Lift clients when changing their position.

    b. Slide clients up in bed every two hours.

    c. Keep the bed clean and dry.

    d. Prevent clients from sliding down in bed.

58. Why are diabetes and cardiovascular diseases risk factors for skin breakdown and delayed healing?

    a. Compromise oxygen delivery to tissues

    b. Create poor tissue perfusion

    c. Cause poor and delayed healing

    d. Cause buildup of glucose in the bloodstream

59. What is an example of wound healing by primary intention?

    a. An open wound

    b. A laceration

    c. A closed surgical wound

    d. A pressure ulcer

60. What function does a scab serve?

    a. Protects the wound from bleeding

    b. Provides something to pick

    c. Keeps drainage off clothing

    d. Serves to aid hemostasis and inhibit contamination

61. What is the most selective method of debridement that causes the least amount of damage to healthy surrounding and healing tissues?

    a. Mechanical

    b. Sharp

    c. Chemical

    d. Autolytic

62. What is larval therapy used for?

    a. Cleanses chronic wounds

    b. Debrides oozing wounds

    c. Removes bacteria

    d. Promotes the use of maggots

63. What are the benefits of semi-occlusive dressings?

    a. Remains moist and can retain a small amount of serous exudates

    b. Does not promote epithelial growth

    c. Slows the healing process

    d. Increases the risk of infection

64. What are Montgomery straps used for?

    a. They replace tape on the skin.

    b. They are replaced less often than taped dressings.

    c. They are used for wounds requiring frequent dressing changes.

    d. They are used for pressure sores.

65. Why is suction used on a wound?

    a. To remove drainage

    b. To promote healing

    c. To speed tissue generation, reduce swelling around the wound, and enhance wound healing

    d. To prevent a scab forming on the wound

66. What is the danger of applying heat to a large localized body area?

    a. Fainting

    b. A drop in blood pressure

    c. Arterial vasodilation

    d. Shivering

67. What is the rebound phenomenon?

    a. Prolonged application of heat or cold causes the reverse action.

    b. Using cold therapy actually promotes vasodilation.

    c. Using heat therapy actually promotes vasoconstriction.

    d. It occurs at the time of the maximum therapeutic effect.

68. What is suppuration?

    a. Wound drainage

    b. Inflammatory response

    c. Client positioning

    d. Pus formation

CHAPTER 25

Perioperative Nursing

KEY TERM REVIEW

Match each term with its appropriate definition.

1. _____ Atelectasis
2. _____ Bier block
3. _____ Circulating nurse
4. _____ Closed-wound
5. _____ Conscious sedation
6. _____ Elective surgery
7. _____ Emergency surgery
8. _____ Epidural anesthesia
9. _____ General anesthesia
10. _____ Intraoperative phase
11. _____ Local anesthesia
12. _____ Nerve block
13. _____ Penrose drain
14. _____ Perioperative period
15. _____ Postoperative phase
16. _____ Preoperative phase
17. _____ Regional anesthesia
18. _____ Scrub person
19. _____ Spinal anesthesia
20. _____ Thrombophlebitis
21. _____ Topical anesthesia

a. Surgery performed immediately to preserve function or the life of the client

b. Also referred to as subarachnoid block (SAB)

c. The assistant to the surgeons, usually a UAP but can be an RN or LPN

d. three phases known as preoperative, intraoperative, and postoperative drainage systems

e. Causes the loss of all sensations and consciousness by blocking awareness centers in the brain

f. The temporary interruption of transmission of nerve impulses to and from a specific area of the brain

g. The collapse of the alveoli, which may result from stagnation of fluid in the lungs

h. An injection into a specific area that is used for minor surgical procedures such as suturing a wound or performing a biopsy

i. Most often used for procedures involving the arm, wrist, or hand with an occlusion tourniquet applied to the extremity to prevent infiltration and absorption of the injected intravenous agent beyond the involved extremity

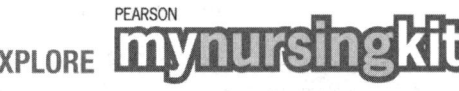

EXPLORE mynursingkit
www.mynursingkit.com

MyNursingKit is your one stop for online chapter review materials and resources. Prepare for success with additional NCLEX®-style practice questions, interactive assignments and activities, web links, animations and videos, and more! Register your access code from the front of your textbook at www.mynursingkit.com

Look for these resources:
- NCLEX® Review
- Case Studies
- Videos and Animations

j. A minimal depression of the level of consciousness in which the client retains the ability to maintain a patent airway and respond appropriately to commands

k. That which is applied directly to the skin and mucous membranes, open skin surfaces, wounds, and burns

l. A drain connected to either an electric suction machine or a portable drainage suction, such as a Hemovac or Jackson-Pratt

m. An injection of an anesthetic agent into the epidural space, the area inside the spinal column but outside the dura mater

n. The phase that begins when the decision to have surgery is made; it ends when the client is transferred to the operating table

o. A drain inserted to permit drainage of excessive serosanguineous fluid and purulent material and to promote healing of underlying tissue

p. The phase that begins when the client is transferred to the operating table and ends when the client is admitted to the postanesthesia care unit (PACU) or the recovery room

q. Surgery performed when surgical intervention is the preferred treatment for a condition that is not imminently life threatening

r. The nurse who coordinates activities and manages client care by continually assessing client safety, aseptic procedures, and the environment

s. An inflammation of a vein followed by formation of a blood clot or emboli (a blood clot that has moved)

t. The phase that begins with the admission of the client to the postanesthesia area and ends when healing is complete

u. A technique in which the anesthetic agent is injected into and around a nerve or small nerve group that supplies sensation to a small area of the body

KEY TOPIC REVIEW

22. List the three phases of surgery.

23. List nursing activities related to the preoperative phase.

24. List three areas where perioperative nursing is practiced.

25. List ways surgical procedures are commonly grouped.

26. List five things that affect the degree of risk involved in a surgical procedure.

27. List things that may affect older adults' healing and responses to medication and surgery.

28. List two things that can increase surgical risks.

29. List four things that a malnourished client is at risk for.

30. List medications that can increase surgical risk.

31. List five things that the surgeon should inform the client about and obtain informed consent from the client or legal guardian.

32. List the new preoperative revised guidelines for elective surgeries.

33. List commonly used preoperative medications.

34. List the three steps for the Universal Protocol for Preventing Wrong Site, Wrong Procedure, Wrong Person Surgery.

35. List the body's response to general anesthesia.

36. List ways that general anesthetics are administered.

37. List eight things that are monitored during surgery.

38. List nine things that maintain the client's safety and help maintain homeostasis.

39. List what the nurse documents during the perioperative plan of care.

40. List objective indicators of pain.

41. List nursing interventions designed to promote client recovery and prevent complications.

42. List six things the nurse assesses the wound for.

CASE STUDY

43. The scrub nurse was preparing the operating room for an arthroplasty of the left knee. Everything was ready for the surgeon, and the client was on his way to the OR. A student nurse was assigned to observe the surgery and was gowning up. The student went into the operating room but no one was there yet. This was the student's first experience in the OR and she was excited about it. She was looking around and bumped into a tray of instruments when one fell on the floor. She knew the items were sterile and she picked it up placing it on a side table. She was about ready to ask the scrub nurse what she should do about it when the client was brought in. The room was extremely busy and everyone she approached did not have time for her. She kept getting pushed back further from the client and from the contaminated instrument.

    1. Why is it important to maintain sterility in the operating room?

    2. Where should the student have waited instead of entering the OR?

    3. How can the student inform them not to use that instrument?

    4. What should the student have done to prevent the client from getting an infection?

REVIEW QUESTIONS

44. What affects a child's ability to cope with the physiologic and psychologic stresses of surgery?

    a. Support group

    b. Reason for surgery (elective vs. emergency)

    c. Age and development

    d. Time of the year, whether in school or out of school

45. What is informed consent?

    a. The client agrees to the procedure.

    b. The client has been informed about what the procedure is.

    c. The client has been informed and involved in decisions affecting his or her health.

    d. The client has given consent.

46. What is the nurse's responsibility with the consent form after the physician has received informed consent?

    a. Send the form to the operating room

    b. May witness the client's signature on the agency consent form

    c. Ensure that the consent form is signed

    d. Answer any questions the client may have

47. What is the overall goal in the preoperative period?

    a. To ensure that the client is mentally and physically prepared for surgery

    b. To premedicate the client

    c. To do an assessment

    d. To keep the family calm

48. When does discharge planning begin for the perioperative client?

    a. When the client is ready to go home

    b. When the client is prepared to participate in the education process

    c. When the client is admitted

    d. When the family is available to participate

49. What is the purpose of hygienic measures?

    a. To cleanse the client because he or she will not be able to shower for several days after surgery

    b. To reduce the risk of wound infection

    c. To remove daily soil from the skin

    d. To reduce the number of bacteria on the skin

50. How do circulating nurses and scrub nurses ensure that no items are left in the client during surgery?

    a. They count all sponges and instruments to ensure nothing is left inside.

    b. They check the surgical site for bumps that don't belong.

    c. The surgeon keeps track of what is used and tells the nurse.

    d. Surgery is videotaped and they can check to make sure nothing was left in the client.

51. How does surgery traumatize the body?

    a. Disrupts protective mechanisms and homeostasis

    b. Disrupts hemostasis

    c. Disrupts urinary system

    d. Disrupts cardiovascular system

52. How should clients be positioned in the OR?

    a. Clients should be positioned with consideration of normal joint range of motion and good body alignment.

    b. Clients should be positioned so the surgical site is easily accessible.

    c. Clients should be comfortable.

    d. Clients should position themselves.

53. Why are nurses so important during the postoperative phase?

    a. They provide care to the client.

    b. They need to monitor the client's vital signs.

    c. Anesthesia impairs the ability of clients to respond to environmental stimuli.

    d. Clients cannot care for themselves and will need to be medicated.

54. Why is an unconscious client positioned on the side during the immediate postanesthetic stage?

    a. Allows drainage of mucus or vomitus out of the mouth

    b. Reduces pressure on the spinal column

    c. Promotes sinus drainage

    d. Helps expand the diaphragm

55. Why is the upper arm supported with a pillow?

    a. To maintain proper alignment

    b. To allow for full expansion of the lungs

    c. To keep it from falling off the gurney

    d. To provide comfort for the client

56. What is the common cause of postoperative hypotension?

    a. A quick change in the position

    b. Too much anesthesia

    c. Hypovolemia due to fluid loss

    d. Excessive IV fluid

57. What does using the incentive spirometer do?

    a. Gives a client the incentive to get well

    b. Measures the lung capacity

    c. Improves lung capacity

    d. Enhances inhalation and ventilation

58. What position permits the greatest lung expansion?

    a. Lying

    b. Standing

    c. Side-lying

    d. Sitting

59. What does wound suction do?

    a. Hastens the healing process

    b. Drains excess exudates

    c. Removes blood

    d. Connects to the inserted drain

CHAPTER 26

SENSORY PERCEPTION

KEY TERM REVIEW

Match each term with its appropriate definition.

1. _____ Acute confusion
2. _____ Awareness
3. _____ Cultural care deprivation
4. _____ Delirium
5. _____ Kinesthetic
6. _____ Sensoristasis
7. _____ Sensory deficit
8. _____ Sensory deprivation
9. _____ Sensory overload
10. _____ Sensory perception
11. _____ Sensory reception
12. _____ Stereognosis

a. The term used to describe when a person is in optimal arousal

b. The ability to perceive and understand an object through touch by its size, shape, and texture

c. The occurrence of a person who experiences excessive sensory input and is unable to process or manage the stimuli

d. The process of receiving stimuli or data

e. A client with a condition that needs care that is directed to promoting orientation to time, place, person, and situation

f. Generally thought of as a decrease in or lack of meaningful stimuli

g. Often called acute confusion which has an abrupt onset and a cause which, when treated, reverses the confusion

h. The impaired reception, perception, or both, of one or more of the senses

i. The ability to perceive environmental stimuli and body reactions and to respond appropriately through thought and action

j. A lack of culturally assistive, supportive, or facilitative acts

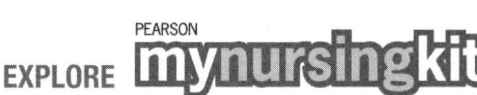

EXPLORE PEARSON mynursingkit

www.mynursingkit.com

MyNursingKit is your one stop for online chapter review materials and resources. Prepare for success with additional NCLEX®-style practice questions, interactive assignments and activities, web links, animations and videos, and more! Register your access code from the front of your textbook at www.mynursingkit.com

Look for these resources:
- NCLEX® Review
- Case Studies
- Videos and Animations

k. The conscious organization and translation of the data or stimuli into meaningful information

l. The awareness of the position and movement of the body parts

KEY TOPIC REVIEW

13. List three things that are essential for an individual's senses.

14. List the two components that the sensory process involves.

15. List four aspects of the sensory process.

16. List the two components of the reticular activating system.

17. List external stimuli.

18. List internal stimuli.

19. List processes of cognition of cerebral functioning.

20. List six things that can contribute to sensory overload.

21. List a number of factors that affect the amount and quality of sensory stimulation.

22. List four ototoxic medications.

23. List the six components from the nursing assessment of sensory-perceptual functioning.

24. List data that significant others can provide about a client's hearing ability.

25. List specific sensory tests performed by nurses during a physical assessment.

26. List signs that indicate social deprivation.

CASE STUDY

27. Jerold was admitted to the hospital after he fell off a ladder. He is 77 years old and lives alone. His wife died 13 years ago and he has been able to care for himself. He has three children who visit at least once a month. He wears glasses and has some problems hearing. He is a retired postal worker and continues to walk daily. The nurse performing the assessment noticed that he seems to be very lonely and talks to all the nurses about moving into an assisted living facility. He feels he will be able to socialize more than he does now. The fall fractured his left tibia and he will have a walking cast on for about six weeks.

    1. Should the nurse contact social services for transferring him to a facility during his recuperation?

    2. What should the nurse assess as far as sensory impairments?

    3. Should the client be discharged to his home?

    4. Should nurses look at a client's age or at the ability to care for self?

REVIEW QUESTIONS

28. What does visceral refer to?

    a. Any large organ within the body

    b. Having to do with the stomach

    c. Dealing with food

    d. Major organs

29. Which of the following diseases restricts blood flow to the receptor organs and the brain?

    a. Arteriosclerosis

    b. Arthrosclerosis

    c. Atherosclerosis

    d. Arteriosclerotic

30. What is the leading cause of blindness in the United States?

    a. Cardiovascular disease

    b. Cerebral vascular accidents

    c. Diabetes insipidus

    d. Diabetes mellitus

31. What places the client at risk for sensory overload?

    a. Insufficient stimuli

    b. External stimuli

    c. Internal stimuli

    d. Excessive stimuli

32. What sound level in the critical care unit can cause sensory overload?

    a. 45 decibels

    b. 60–83 decibels

    c. 50–65 decibels

    d. 40–60 decibels

33. What must a nurse consider to provide for continuity of care?

    a. The client's needs for assistance with care in the home or residential treatment setting

    b. The client's understanding of his or her needs when discharged

    c. The client's ability to perform all ADLs without help

    d. What the client could do when admitted and any changes in their ability to care for themselves

34. Why should pregnant women be advised of the importance of testing for syphilis and rubella?

    a. STIs can be transmitted to her sexual partners.

    b. They could be transferred to the fetus.

    c. They can cause hearing impairments in newborns.

    d. They could cause visual impairments in the newborn.

35. What should nurses do when assisting clients who have a sensory deficit?

    a. Promote the use of other senses.

    b. Provide them with stimulating activities.

    c. Talk loudly when addressing the client.

    d. Encourage client safety.

36. What does a person with a visual impairment who is unable to observe most nonverbal cues during communication rely on?

    a. Other senses

    b. The spoken word and tone of voice

    c. A seeing-eye dog

    d. Phrasing of the message

37. How does a loss of vision affect a person's quality of life?

    a. Increased disability

    b. Decreased depression

    c. More autonomy

    d. Becoming independent of others

38. When caring for a client with a visual impairment, what should nurses do when entering the room?

    a. Speak loudly

    b. Turn on the lights

    c. Knock on the door

    d. Announce themselves

39. When dealing with a confused client, what is the most important answer to help with orientation?

    a. Identify time and place.

    b. Wear a name tag.

    c. Introduce yourself.

    d. Ask the client's name and where he or she is.

40. What should nurses do to stimulate an unconscious client?

    a. Keep the room quiet.

    b. Play loud music.

    c. Talk normally to the client.

    d. Wait until the client wakes up.

CHAPTER 27

SELF-CONCEPT

KEY TERM REVIEW

Match each term with its appropriate definition.

1. _____ Body image
2. _____ Core self-concept
3. _____ Global self
4. _____ Global self-esteem
5. _____ Ideal self
6. _____ Role ambiguity
7. _____ Role conflicts
8. _____ Role development
9. _____ Role mastery
10. _____ Role performance
11. _____ Role strain
12. _____ Self-awareness
13. _____ Self-concept
14. _____ Self-esteem
15. _____ Specific self-esteem

a. Relates what a person in a particular role does to the behaviors expected of that role

b. The relationship between one's perception of self and others' perception of him or her

c. The image of physical self or how a person perceives the size, appearance, and functions of the body and its parts

d. How much one approves of a certain part of oneself

e. Frustration due to feelings because they are made to feel inadequate or unsuited to a role

f. The beliefs and images that are most vital to a person's identity, and how they perceive and evaluate themselves

g. Socialization into a particular role

h. The collective beliefs and images one holds about oneself

i. One's judgment of one's own worth

j. A person's self-perception of how they would like to be

k. How much one likes oneself as a whole

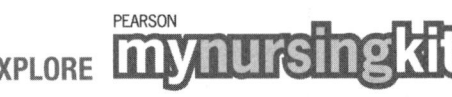

EXPLORE PEARSON **mynursingkit**

www.mynursingkit.com

MyNursingKit is your one stop for online chapter review materials and resources. Prepare for success with additional NCLEX®-style practice questions, interactive assignments and activities, web links, animations and videos, and more! Register your access code from the front of your textbook at www.mynursingkit.com

Look for these resources:
- NCLEX® Review
- Case Studies
- Videos and Animations

l. When expectations are unclear, and people do not know what to do, or how to do it, and are unable to predict the reactions of others to their behavior

m. The person's behaviors meet social expectations

n. One's mental image of oneself

o. Problems that arise from opposing or incompatible expectations

KEY TOPIC REVIEW

16. List five things that influence self-concept.

17. List four dimensions of self-concept.

18. List five things involved in introspection.

19. List eight areas that people are thought to base their self-concepts on.

20. List four components of self-concept.

21. List eight ways people view their identity.

22. List four affective sensations of the body.

23. List an individual's perception of how one should behave.

24. List three influences on the nurse's self-concept.

25. List four things included in personal identity.

26. List three broad steps in the development of one's self-concept.

27. List things that a person with a strong sense of identity has.

28. List eight things included in body image.

29. List six roles that a person might have.

30. List external resources.

31. List ways people respond to stressors.

32. List eight guidelines for conducting a psychosocial assessment.

CASE STUDY

33. Reeja moved here from India three years ago. She received her nursing degree while in India and she sat for the NCLEX® test and passed it in the United States. Her first experience here was in a large city hospital working with children. She was not given a preceptor and was left to learn on her own. Because she was from a different country and culture, other nurses were not very friendly to her nor did they help her when she got bogged down with her clients. Her English was good but she did have a thick accent and tried very hard to overcome it. She strived to be friendly and offered help to all the other nurses. After about six months, she decided to try another hospital and was hired in a medical–surgical unit where she was given a preceptor.

The staff members have been very friendly and helpful. It is much easier for her at this hospital and no one seems to mind that she is from India. She has a husband and two children with the third one on the way. She likes living in the United States, but feels some people are unfriendly to foreigners. She has a hard time explaining to her husband and children why she was so unhappy and had to change jobs.

1. What would her self-concept be like through this ordeal?
2. How could the failure from the first position affect her self-esteem?
3. Would her self-concept in the first position be due to role strain?
4. If nurses treat other nurses from other countries this badly, how will they be able to deal therapeutically with clients from different cultural backgrounds?

REVIEW QUESTIONS

34. How does a person get a self-concept?
    a. The person is born with it.
    b. It comes from the person's parents.
    c. It develops as a result of social interactions with others.
    d. It develops from family and culture.

35. How often does a person maintain and evaluate a self-concept?
    a. Occasionally
    b. Weekly
    c. Yearly
    d. Continuously

36. When can low self-esteem result?
    a. When there is a discrepancy between ideal self and perceived self
    b. When the discrepancy is great between ideal self and perceived self
    c. When there is no discrepancy between ideal self and perceived self
    d. Only when a person is depressed

37. Why is each person's self-concept like a piece of art?
    a. It's a work in progress.
    b. It starts with a blank canvas.
    c. At the center of the art are the beliefs and images that are most vital to the person's identity.
    d. Our self-concept is developed through our contact with friends and family members.

38. What does having a basic self-concept include?
    a. How we see ourselves and how we are seen by others
    b. How we think others see us
    c. How we want others to see us
    d. How others think they see us

39. What can role conflict lead to?

    a. Internal unrest

    b. Less tension

    c. Increase in self-esteem

    d. Embarrassment if needs for achievement, independence, and recognition are unmet

40. What influences a young child's values?

    a. Family and culture

    b. Peers

    c. Teachers

    d. Neighbors

41. How can nurses help clients who have an altered self-concept?

    a. Provide them with hope for their illness.

    b. Establish a nontherapeutic relationship.

    c. Assist clients to evaluate themselves and make behavioral changes.

    d. Guide them to develop an improved self-concept.

42. What can change the level of self-concept over time?

    a. Personality changes

    b. Maturation

    c. Events

    d. Aging

43. What is personal identity?

    a. The conscious sense of individuality and uniqueness that is continually evolving throughout life

    b. The sense of identity that provides a person with a feeling of continuity

    c. What a person thinks he or she is

    d. The name on a driver's license

44. What are the two aspects of body image?

    a. Psychosocial and physical

    b. Psychologic and personal

    c. Cognitive and affective

    d. Physical and personal

45. What concern about body image does an adolescent have?

    a. Cultural standards

    b. Healthy habits

    c. Media-portrayed ideal body

    d. Name brand clothing

CHAPTER 28

SEXUALITY

KEY TERM REVIEW

Match each term with its appropriate definition.

1. _____ Androgyny
2. _____ Cross-dresser
3. _____ Desire phase
4. _____ Dissatisfaction
5. _____ Dyspareunia
6. _____ Excitement phase
7. _____ Female orgasmic disorder
8. _____ Female sexual arousal disorder
9. _____ Gender-role behavior
10. _____ Genital intercourse
11. _____ Hypoactive sexual desire disorder
12. _____ Intersex
13. _____ Male erectile disorder
14. _____ Male orgasmic disorder
15. _____ Orgasmic phase
16. _____ Resolution phase
17. _____ Sexual aversion disorder

a. The sexual problems more commonly related to the emotional problems of the relationship than to the physiologic responses; a lack of fulfillment

b. How one values oneself as a sexual being

c. A common form of sexual activity for heterosexual couples which can be both physically and emotionally satisfying

d. The integration of the somatic, emotional, intellectual, and social aspects of sexual being, in ways that are positively enriching and that enhance personality, communication, and love

e. The outward expression of a person's sense of maleness or femaleness as well as the expression of what is perceived as gender-appropriate behavior

f. Severe pain caused only on touch or attempted vaginal entry

g. Flexibility in gender roles in the belief that most characteristics and behaviors are human qualities that should not be limited to one specific gender or the other

h. Biologically speaking there are many gradations running from female to male, and in some cases the gender is clear, in others there is a blending of both genders within the same individual, and in some it is unclear

18. _____ Sexual health
19. _____ Sexual orientation
20. _____ Sexual self-concept
21. _____ Transgenderism
22. _____ Transsexuals
23. _____ Vaginismus
24. _____ Vestibulitis
25. _____ Vulvodynia

i. Constant, unremitting burning that is localized to the vulva with an acute onset

j. The onset of pain during or immediately after intercourse which can be experienced by both women and men

k. The response cycle that starts in the brain with conscious sexual desires

l. A condition called gender dysphoria, when one has a strong and persistent feeling of discomfort with one's assigned gender

m. The involuntary spasm of the outer one third of the vaginal muscles, making penetration of the vagina painful and sometimes impossible

n. A deficiency or absence of sexual fantasies and persistent low interest or a total lack of interest in sexual activity

o. The condition in which there are contradictions among chromosomal gender, gonad gender, internal organs, and external genital appearance

p. Typically males who want to express the feminine side of their personality who are not interested in permanently altering their bodies through surgical means

q. The lack of vaginal lubrication, which causes pain and discomfort during intercourse

r. Two primary physiologic changes: the increase of blood flow to various parts of the body resulting in the erection of the penis and clitoris, and swelling of the labia, testes, and breasts

s. When the sexual response stops before an orgasm occurs

t. The extreme difficulty of ejaculation

u. A man who usually has erection problems during 25% or more of his sexual interactions

v. One's attraction to people of the same sex, other sex, or both sexes

w. The involuntary climax of sexual tension, accompanied by physiologic and psychologic release

x. A severe distaste for sexual activity, or the thought of sexual activity, which leads to a phobic avoidance of sex

y. The period of return to the unaroused state, which may last 10 to 15 minutes after orgasm, or longer if there is no orgasm

KEY TOPIC REVIEW

26. List three factors that influence a person's sexuality and lead to the wide range of attitudes and behaviors seen in humans.

27. List subtle signs of impending menstruation.

28. List six treatments used for menstrual cramping and pain.

29. List factual information that nurses should discuss with teenagers.

30. List six of the various methods of birth control.

31. List six ways an older adult may define sexuality.

32. List ways that the World Health Organization defines sexual health.

33. List five critical components of sexual health.

34. List five things that can change an individual's appearance and function affecting body image.

35. List things that influence gender-role behavior.

36. List things that sexually healthy people are ethically motivated to do.

37. List four sexual varieties.

38. List four contradictions with intersex babies.

39. List five things that being transgendered puts women and men at extreme risk of being.

40. List six varieties of sexuality.

41. List five factors that can influence a person's sexuality.

42. List five diseases that have sexual side effects.

CASE STUDY

43. Roger, a 17-year-old male, has been having sex with several of his classmates. He has been experiencing itching and drainage from his penis. He was afraid to talk to his parents, so he looked for a free clinic where he could get checked out. One of the girls he was with complained of a sore throat and asked Roger if he was ill. He told her no since he did not think her symptoms had anything to do with him. Another girl confided in her mother that she had missed her menstrual cycle and was having vaginal itching and a foul-smelling discharge.

    1. What do you think Roger's problem is?
    2. Is there a correlation with the girl's sore throat?
    3. When he goes to the clinic, what is their responsibility to protect the public?
    4. What problems does the second girl have?

REVIEW QUESTIONS

44. What is human sexuality?

    a. The gender differences between male and female

    b. Procreation to expand the human race

    c. An individual personal phenomenon evolving from life experiences

    d. Attitudes and behaviors seen in humans

45. How is a "normal" sexual expression described?

    a. Whatever behaviors give pleasure and satisfaction to those adults involved

    b. An expression of love between consenting adults

    c. A sexual expression accepted by societal standards

    d. Normal universal sexual behaviors

46. When does the development of sexuality begin?

    a. During puberty

    b. At conception and throughout the life span

    c. Between the ages of 10 and 13

    d. After birth

47. What causes dysmenorrhea?

    a. Secondary sex characteristics

    b. Postmenstrual complications

    c. Toxic shock syndrome

    d. Powerful uterine contractions

48. What are the most common bacterial infections among adolescents?

    a. Meningitis

    b. Strep throat

    c. STIs

    d. Jock itch

49. How is a person's degree of sexual health best determined?

    a. By the individual

    b. By the sexual partner

    c. By a professional

    d. By age

50. What enables people to form intimate relationships throughout life?

    a. Negative sexual self-concept

    b. Positive sexual self-concept

    c. Neutral sexual self-concept

    d. Heterosexual self-concept

51. What does sexual health include?

    a. Ability to maintain a relationship

    b. Age-related activities

    c. Both freedom and responsibilities

    d. Consenting adults

52. What are people who are attracted to both genders referred to as?

    a. Homosexual

    b. Heterosexual

    c. Gay or lesbian

    d. Bisexual

53. What does the author consider the ongoing love affair that each of us has with ourselves throughout our lifetime?

    a. Masturbation

    b. Sexual relationships

    c. Body image

    d. Eroticism

54. What is the most common cause of sexual aversion?

    a. Childhood sexual abuse or adult rape

    b. Parents who are abusive

    c. Parents who do not demonstrate love

    d. Cultures that only use sex for procreation

55. What is the real goal of being sexual?

    a. Frustration

    b. Mutual pleasuring and intimacy

    c. Anxiety

    d. Procreation

56. What is one of the most common sexual dysfunctions among men?

    a. Homosexuality

    b. Frigidity

    c. Premature ejaculation

    d. Rapid ejaculation

57. What do women use that increases their chances of acquiring toxic shock syndrome?

    a. Sanitary pads

    b. Tampons

    c. Colored underwear

    d. Tight jeans

58. What medications do men take that can slow their ejaculation?

    a. Antibiotics

    b. Antidepressants

    c. Antiemetics

    d. Antacids

CHAPTER 29

SPIRITUALITY

KEY TERM REVIEW

Match each term with its appropriate definition.

1. _____ Agnostic
2. _____ Atheist
3. _____ Faith
4. _____ Holy day
5. _____ Hope
6. _____ Kosher
7. _____ Meditation
8. _____ Monotheism
9. _____ Polytheism
10. _____ Prayer
11. _____ Presencing
12. _____ Spiritual distress
13. _____ Spiritual health
14. _____ Spirituality
15. _____ Transcendence

a. The belief in more than one God

b. The part of being human that seeks meaningfulness through inter-, intra-, and transpersonal connection

c. The human communication with divine and spiritual entities

d. The food prepared according to Jewish law

e. The act of being present, being there, or just being with a client

f. To believe in or be committed to something or someone

g. A person who doubts the existence of God or a supreme being or believes the existence of God has not been proved

h. The capacity to reach out beyond oneself to extend oneself beyond personal concerns and to take on broader life perspectives, activities, and purposes

i. A day set aside for special religious observance

j. A challenge to the well-being or to the belief system that provides strength, meaning, and hope to life

k. A concept that incorporates spirituality

EXPLORE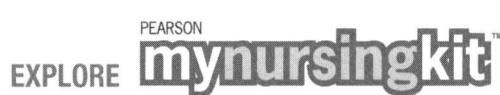

www.mynursingkit.com

MyNursingKit is your one stop for online chapter review materials and resources. Prepare for success with additional NCLEX®-style practice questions, interactive assignments and activities, web links, animations and videos, and more! Register your access code from the front of your textbook at www.mynursingkit.com

Look for these resources:
- NCLEX® Review
- Case Studies
- Videos and Animations

l. A feeling of being generally alive, purposeful, and fulfilled

m. The belief in the existence of one God

n. Focusing one's thoughts or engaging in self-reflection or contemplation

o. A person without belief in God

KEY TOPIC REVIEW

16. List the aspects of spirituality.

17. List four factors that influence spirit titer.

18. List four manifestations of spiritual health, as defined by the Nursing Outcomes Classification project.

19. List four ways we can relate to our inner self.

20. List four physiologic problems that can challenge spiritual well-being.

21. List six factors related to treatment for physiologic problems.

22. List things that define spiritual wellness according to Pilch.

23. List three ways that the expression of a person's spiritual energy to others is manifested in loving relationships with and in service to others.

24. List things the organized religions offer.

25. List five events that are related to traditional religious practices.

26. List the guidelines for nurses that were offered by Winslow and Winslow (2003).

27. List three things included on high holy days.

28. List six examples of sacred symbols that carry spiritual significance.

29. List four reasons why sacred symbols are worn.

30. List different types of prayer experience.

31. List questions a nurse must consider before sharing personal beliefs.

32. List examples of orderliness in the universe.

CASE STUDY

33. Martin, a 42-year-old male, was admitted to the hospital for a coronary bypass and mitral valve repair. He came in with a male friend and said he was divorced and had three children. He is unemployed because of his heart problems but plans on returning to his job as an accountant after his rehabilitation. When asked about his spiritual needs, he stated he had not attended church in five years. He wears a cross neck chain and filled out Catholic as his religion. Martin's parents died from heart problems when they were in their 40s and he is worried that he will also die young. His support system is limited and the nurse is concerned about him and feels he should talk with his clergy.

   1. Does illness bring out spirituality in a person?
   2. What does he have to focus on to make his life worth living?
   3. How can talking to a clergy improve his chances for survival?
   4. What can the nurse's presence do to assist the client's spirituality?

REVIEW QUESTIONS

34. What can meeting the client's spiritual needs do?

    a. Decrease suffering and aid in physical and mental healing

    b. Increase suffering and help psychologically

    c. Impair physical mobility

    d. Reduce the need for medications

35. What happens when the spirit titer is low?

    a. Inspiration

    b. Depression

    c. Regression

    d. Aggression

36. What questions might a client with a terminal illness without spiritual beliefs ask?

    a. Is there really a God?

    b. How can a just God allow people to suffer?

    c. Why me?

    d. If I believe, will it change the outcome?

37. What is religion?

    a. A belief system

    b. The reason we exist

    c. A way to make money

    d. An organized system of beliefs and practices

38. Where do religious rules of conduct come from?

    a. Cultural influences

    b. The Bible

    c. Sunday school

    d. Society

39. What happens when a client no longer has hope?

    a. The illness progresses.

    b. The client gives up trying.

    c. The client's spirituality is decreased.

    d. It promotes fear.

40. What will help nurses to converse therapeutically with clients?

    a. Understanding cultural differences

    b. Using the client's language for spirituality

    c. Following the same belief system

    d. Checking the client's history for religion preferences

41. How many times a day do Muslims follow the practice of prayer?

    a. Four

    b. Three

    c. Two

    d. Five

42. What religions practice the Sabbath on Saturday?

    a. Jews and Muslims

    b. Catholics and Lutherans

    c. Jews and Seventh-Day Adventists

    d. Christians and Jews

43. What religious group does not allow blood transfusions?

    a. Muslims

    b. Jews

    c. Jehovah's Witnesses

    d. Christians

44. What organization mandates that each client admitted to an institution's care must be assessed for spiritual beliefs and practices?

    a. JCAHO

    b. NLN

    c. ANA

    d. OSHA

45. What is the value of prayer?

    a. Provides an outlet

    b. Involves a sense of love and connection

    c. Provides the ability to express care

    d. Provides a sense of security and connectivity

46. What is the nurse's major responsibility when a client wants to pray?

    a. Lead the group.

    b. Call for clergy.

    c. Provide privacy.

    d. Schedule prayer when care is not needed.

47. What may be necessary when the nurse makes a diagnosis of spiritual distress?

    a. Clergy

    b. Referrals

    c. Physician's order

    d. A second opinion

CHAPTER 30

COPING WITH STRESS, LOSS, AND DEATH

KEY TERM REVIEW

Match each term with its appropriate definition.

1. _____ Algor mortis
2. _____ Anticipatory grief
3. _____ Anticipatory loss
4. _____ Anxiety
5. _____ Bereavement
6. _____ Burnout
7. _____ Caregiver burden
8. _____ Cerebral death
9. _____ Closed awareness
10. _____ Complicated grief
11. _____ Coping
12. _____ Coping strategy
13. _____ Crisis counseling
14. _____ Crisis intervention
15. _____ Ego defense
16. _____ Fear
17. _____ General adaptation
18. _____ Liver mortis
19. _____ Mourning
20. _____ Mutual pretense

a. A loss experienced by one person but cannot be verified by others

b. The behavioral process through which grief is eventually resolved or altered; often influenced by culture, custom, and spiritual beliefs

c. A natural or learned way of responding to a changing environment or specific problems or situations

d. Any event or stimulus that causes an individual to experience stress

e. The focus on solving immediate problems which involves individual groups or families

f. Advanced emotional experiences such as the wife who grieves before her husband dies

g. An emotion or feeling of apprehension aroused by impending or seeming changes, pain, or another perceived threat

h. The gradual decrease of the body's temperature after death

i. Unhealthy grief that exists when strategies to cope with the loss are maladaptive

j. The stiffening of the body that occurs 2 to 4 hours after death

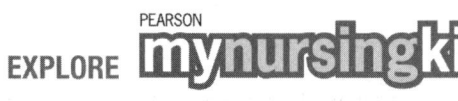

EXPLORE **mynursingkit** PEARSON

www.mynursingkit.com

MyNursingKit is your one stop for online chapter review materials and resources. Prepare for success with additional NCLEX®-style practice questions, interactive assignments and activities, web links, animations and videos, and more! Register your access code from the front of your textbook at www.mynursingkit.com

Look for these resources:
- NCLEX® Review
- Case Studies
- Videos and Animations

21. _____ Open awareness
22. _____ Palliative care
23. _____ Perceived loss
24. _____ Rigor mortis
25. _____ Stressor

k. A loss experienced before the loss actually occurs

l. A discoloration appearing in the lowermost or dependent areas of the body

m. The client and others know about the impending death and feel comfortable discussing it, even though it is difficult

n. A state of mental uneasiness, apprehension, dread, foreboding, or a feeling of helplessness relating to an impending or anticipated threat

o. An acute state of intense psychologic sadness and suffering experienced after the tragic loss of a loved one

p. The ability to deal with change

q. A complex syndrome of behavior that can be likened to the exhaustion stage of the general adaptation syndrome, manifesting physical and emotional depletion

r. The occurrence when the higher brain center, the cerebral cortex, is irreversibly destroyed

s. Unconscious psychologic adaptive mechanisms or mental mechanisms that develop as the personality attempts to defend itself, establish compromises among conflicting impulses, and calm inner tensions

t. A short-term helping process to assist clients to work their crisis to its resolution or to restore their precrisis level of functioning

u. Stress response characterized by a chain or pattern of physiologic events

v. A situation where the client is not made aware of impending death

w. Stress that produces responses such as chronic fatigue, sleeping difficulties, and high blood pressure

x. An approach that improves the quality of life of clients and their families facing the problems associated with life-threatening illness, through the prevention and relief of suffering, by means of early identification and impeccable assessment and treatment of pain, and other problems such as physical, psychosocial, and spiritual

y. The client, family, and health personnel know the prognosis is terminal but do not talk about it and make an effort not to raise the subject

KEY TOPIC REVIEW

26. List three responses when a person faces stresses.

27. List the four kinds of stressors.

28. List five consequences of stress.

29. List three main models of stress.

30. List three parts of the body particularly affected by stress.

144 CHAPTER 30 / Coping with Stress, Loss, and Death

31. List three indicators of stress.

32. List psychologic manifestations of stress.

33. List the four levels of anxiety and how they can be manifested.

34. List the four differences between anxiety and fear.

35. List the extreme feelings of depression.

36. List emotional symptoms of depression.

37. List seven behavioral signs of depression.

38. List five physical signs of depression.

39. List two types of coping strategies.

40. List examples of short-term strategies.

41. List three approaches to coping.

42. List factors that affect the effectiveness of an individual's coping.

43. List two things nurses assess about clients' stress and coping patterns.

44. List 10 symptoms that can accompany grief.

CASE STUDY

45. Helen, a 69-year-old female who has been married for 49 years, retired with her husband to travel and spend more time together. After the first year of retirement, her husband became ill and needed constant care and monitoring. Helen became very depressed and started resenting her husband and the fact that they were stuck at home. As the problems worsened, she also became ill and had no desire to do anything. Her husband had major surgery and afterwards seemed to improve, but then he got worse. He was readmitted for more surgery and lapsed into a coma and died. Helen's depression deepened and she blamed herself for her husband's death. Her physician increased her medication and added sleeping pills, but she continued to stay up at night and would nap during the day. About a week after the funeral she was admitted to the psychiatric unit.

    1. What form of depression is Helen suffering from?

    2. What type of depression is caused from the loss of a loved one?

    3. Could the doctor provide additional help besides medications?

    4. What will nurses be able to provide to improve Helen's situation?

REVIEW QUESTIONS

46. What kind of stressors originate within a person such as an infection or feelings of depression?

    a. External

    b. Internal

    c. Developmental

    d. Situational

47. What kind of stress can be positive or negative and may include death of a loved one, marriage, divorce, birth of a child, or a new job?

    a. Developmental

    b. External

    c. Internal

    d. Situational

48. What stress model may increase the individual's vulnerability to illness?

    a. Stimulus based

    b. Response based

    c. Transaction based

    d. Developmental based

49. What changes the degree of stress an event presents?

    a. Type of event

    b. Time of the event

    c. Individuality

    d. Support system

50. When does the stress syndrome, or GAS, occur in the body?

    a. As soon as stress occurs

    b. After stress has occurred

    c. With the release of certain adaptive hormones

    d. With fight or flight hormones

51. What do the physiologic signs and symptoms of stress result from?

    a. Activation of the sympathetic and neuroendocrine systems

    b. Release of adaptive hormones

    c. Physiologic changes

    d. Psychologic changes

52. What is a common reaction to stress?

    a. Depression

    b. Anxiety

    c. Gastritis

    d. Fear

CHAPTER 30 / Coping with Stress, Loss, and Death

53. Why is anger considered a positive emotion and a sign of emotional maturity?

    a. It is a subjective feeling.

    b. It is an objective feeling.

    c. Growth and beneficial interactions result from it.

    d. It can cause a feeling of guilt.

54. What can verbally expressed anger lead to?

    a. Hostility

    b. Aggression

    c. Antagonism

    d. Destructiveness and violence

55. Why is it beneficial to get anger out into the open?

    a. To clear the air

    b. To be constructive

    c. To identify the source

    d. To clarify the problem

56. What type of depression is a cause for concern and may require treatment?

    a. Prolonged depression

    b. Short-term depression

    c. Developmental depression

    d. Situational depression

57. What are defense mechanisms?

    a. Precursors to physical coping mechanisms

    b. The unconscious mind working to protect the person from anxiety

    c. Increased tension

    d. Adaptive uses

58. What is thinking through the threatening situation, using specific steps to arrive at a solution?

    a. Structuring

    b. Analyzing

    c. Critical thinking

    d. Problem solving

59. What strategies for dealing with clients' anger should nurses employ?

    a. Know and understand your own response to the feelings and expressions of anger.

    b. Do not try to understand the meaning of the client's anger.

    c. Never ask the client what contributed to the anger.

    d. Talk to the client about the anger.

60. What should a nurse do when there is a concern for his or her own safety while working with an angry client?

    a. Put distance between them.

    b. Discharge the client.

    c. Withdraw from the situation.

    d. Maintain support for the individual.

61. Why is it important for nurses to understand the significance of loss?

    a. Because they will also suffer a loss in their lives

    b. To develop the ability to assist clients working through the grieving process

    c. Because they need to be all things to all people

    d. To be able to provide supportive care

62. What is the most upsetting phase for the grieving person facing the loss?

    a. Bargaining

    b. Anger

    c. Confrontation

    d. Accommodation

63. What religion prefers cremation?

    a. Catholics

    b. Muslims

    c. Hindus

    d. Mormons

64. What is the last sense that is considered to be lost?

    a. Smelling

    b. Seeing

    c. Tasting

    d. Hearing

CHAPTER 31

ACTIVITY, EXERCISE, AND SLEEP

KEY TERM REVIEW

Match each term with its appropriate definition.

1. _____ Active ROM exercises
2. _____ Activity tolerance
3. _____ Atrophy
4. _____ Basal metabolic rate
5. _____ Biological rhythms
6. _____ Contracture
7. _____ Functional strength
8. _____ Hypersomnia
9. _____ Hypertrophy
10. _____ Insomnia
11. _____ Log rolling
12. _____ Mobility
13. _____ Narcolepsy
14. _____ NREM sleep
15. _____ Parasomnia
16. _____ Passive ROM exercises
17. _____ Polysomnography
18. _____ Proprioception
19. _____ Range of motion

a. A type of sleep known as non-rapid-eye-movement
b. The ability of the body to perform work and is another goal of exercise
c. Holding the breath and straining against a closed glottis
d. A type of sleep known as rapid-eye-movement
e. The proper standing position with crutches
f. The value of maintaining joint flexibility when another person moves each of the client's joints through its complete range of movement, maximally stretching all muscle groups within each plane over each joint
g. A wasting of the body or of an organ or part
h. Isotonic exercises in which the client moves each joint in the body through its complete range of motion, maximally stretching all muscle groups, within each plane over the joint
i. A term used to describe awareness of posture, movement, and changes in equilibrium and the knowledge of position, weight, and resistance of objects in relation to the body
j. The study of sleep

20. _____ REM sleep
21. _____ Sleep apnea
22. _____ Sleep architecture
23. _____ Sleep hygiene
24. _____ Somnology
25. _____ Tripod position
26. _____ Valsalva maneuver

k. The minimal amount of energy required to sustain life in the waking state

l. The muscles permanently shorten, and the joint becomes fixed in a flexed position

m. The condition when affected individuals obtain sufficient sleep at night but still cannot stay awake during the day

n. A term referring to interventions used to promote sleep

o. The type and amount of exercise or daily living activities an individual is able to perform without experiencing adverse effects

p. The basic organization of normal sleep

q. The control from within the body synchronized with environmental factors, such as light and darkness

r. The inability to fall asleep or remain asleep

s. With strenuous exercise, the muscles enlarge and the efficiency of muscular contraction increases

t. A technique used to turn a client whose body must at all times be kept in straight alignment

u. The maximum range of movement possible for that joint

v. The ability to move freely, easily, rhythmically, and purposefully in the environment

w. A disorder of excessive daytime sleepiness caused by lack of the chemical hypocretin in the area of the central nervous system that regulates sleep

x. A disorder characterized by frequent short breathing pauses during sleep

y. Behavior that may interfere with sleep and may even occur during sleep

z. When an electroencephalogram, electromyogram, and electro-oculogram are recorded simultaneously

KEY TOPIC REVIEW

27. List two predictors of longevity.

28. List four basic elements for coordinated muscle activity and neurologic integration.

29. List three things that posture reflects.

30. List four things that proper body alignment enhances.

31. List four things that determine ROM.

32. List things that isotonic exercises increase.

33. List areas that isometric exercises strengthen.

34. List things that exercise does.

35. List three things that are enhanced due to increased oxygen to the brain.

36. List changes that occur during the aging process.

37. List three things that influence physical activity.

38. List 12 potentially motivating factors for activities.

39. List five systems that are affected by any disorder impairing mobility and activity tolerance.

40. List data pertaining to the problems of immobility that nurses assess.

41. List five ways to prevent clot formation in deep leg veins.

42. List examples of overall goals for clients with actual or potential problems related to mobility or activity.

43. List five of the most common injuries among health care workers.

44. List the major muscle groups that the nurse uses to prevent back strain.

45. List three things that can contribute to hip flexion contractures and low back strain and pain.

46. List symptoms of postural (orthostatic) hypotension.

47. List six reasons we require sleep.

48. List eight causes for psychologic disturbances from the loss of REM sleep.

CASE STUDY

49. Sue, a 56-year-old female nurse, was admitted to the hospital for a knee replacement. She was injured on the job. While running to assist with a code, she slipped on the floor where someone spilled water. Sue's knee hit the edge of a chair and destroyed the joint that was already damaged with osteoarthritis. After the surgery she was sent to an orthopedic joint center to recuperate. She also has problems with her other joints and has problems turning and positioning herself in bed. The knee has a large dressing with a Hemovac drain and ice packs to minimize the swelling. She will be on bed rest for 12 hours and then they will start her on therapy. She normally has problems sleeping and stays awake watching TV.

    1. What will her nurse need to do to ensure good body alignment?

    2. What can her nurse do to protect Sue from injury when turning and positioning?

    3. What can be done to provide comfort for Sue's other joints while on bed rest?

    4. Why does Sue need to sleep?

REVIEW QUESTIONS

50. What can prevent and even reverse many of the chronic diseases experienced by aging adults?

    a. Vitamins

    b. Anti-aging creams

    c. Exercise

    d. Low-carbohydrate diet

51. What groups of women have the lowest mortality rates?

    a. Thin and active

    b. Obese and sedentary

    c. Thin and sedentary

    d. Obese and active

52. What is an essential part of living?

    a. Exercise

    b. Nutrition

    c. Mobility

    d. Activity

53. What does the cerebral cortex operate?

    a. Muscles

    b. Posture

    c. Motor activities

    d. Movement

54. How is bone density and strength maintained?

    a. Calcium supplements

    b. Vitamin D

    c. Milk products

    d. Weight bearing

55. What system suffers the most from prolonged immobility?

    a. Gastrointestinal

    b. Respiratory

    c. Musculoskeletal

    d. Cardiovascular

56. What does bed rest do for clients with medical conditions?

    a. Allows them to heal

    b. Provides rest for the body

    c. Causes complications

    d. Improves overall health

57. How do nurses prevent the complications of immobility?

    a. Get clients out of bed every shift.

    b. Identify clients at risk.

    c. Assess activity level.

    d. Record baseline data.

58. What is the term used to describe the efficient, coordinated, and safe use of the body to move objects and carry out the activities of daily living?

    a. Body mechanics

    b. Ambulating

    c. Mobility

    d. Repositioning

59. How does a person enlarge the base of support?

    a. Bend the knees.

    b. Move the front foot forward.

    c. Keep the item close to the body.

    d. Use the thigh muscles.

60. What is the position of choice for people who have difficulty breathing and for some people with heart problems?

    a. Supine

    b. Prone

    c. Trendelenburg's

    d. Fowler's

61. What position may not be recommended for people with problems of the cervical or lumbar spine?

    a. Supine

    b. Prone

    c. Side-lying

    d. Fowler's

62. What position is good for resting and sleeping clients?

    a. Supine

    b. Prone

    c. Fowler's

    d. Lateral

63. What position should be used for unconscious clients to facilitate drainage from the mouth and prevent aspiration of fluids?

    a. Sims'

    b. Prone

    c. Supine

    d. Lateral

64. What is involved with the sleep–wake cycle?

    a. Cerebral cortex

    b. Cerebellum

    c. Reticular activating system

    d. Growth hormones

65. What is considered to be the number one cause of short-term sleeping difficulties?

    a. Anxiety

    b. Shift work

    c. Light

    d. Stress

66. What is the major goal for clients with sleep disturbances?

    a. Maintain a sleeping pattern.

    b. Get eight hours of sleep a day.

    c. Enhance well-being.

    d. Provide a diversion.

CHAPTER 32

NUTRITION

KEY TERM REVIEW

Match each term with its appropriate definition.

1. _____ Anabolism
2. _____ Basal metabolic rate
3. _____ Body mass index
4. _____ Catabolism
5. _____ Disaccharides
6. _____ Enteral
7. _____ Essential amino acids
8. _____ Fats
9. _____ Glycerides
10. _____ Glycogen
11. _____ Glycogenesis
12. _____ Kilocalorie
13. _____ Kilocoule
14. _____ Lipids
15. _____ Mid-arm circumference
16. _____ Monosaccharides
17. _____ Monounsaturated fatty acid
18. _____ Overnutrition

a. Lipids that are solid at room temperature
b. The process by which glycogen is formed
c. A caloric intake in excess of daily energy requirements resulting in storage of energy in the form of adipose tissue
d. The building of tissue
e. An acid with one double bond
f. An acid that all the carbon atoms are filled to capacity with hydrogen
g. Organic substances that are greasy and insoluble in water but soluble in alcohol or ether
h. Substance with three fatty acids that accounts for 90% of lipids found in food and the body
i. An indicator of changes in body fat stores and whether a person's weight is appropriate for height
j. The breaking down of tissue
k. Sugars which may be double molecules
l. The rate of energy utilization in the body required to maintain essential activities such as breathing

EXPLORE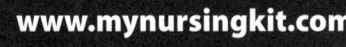

www.mynursingkit.com

MyNursingKit is your one stop for online chapter review materials and resources. Prepare for success with additional NCLEX®-style practice questions, interactive assignments and activities, web links, animations and videos, and more! Register your access code from the front of your textbook at www.mynursingkit.com

Look for these resources:
- NCLEX® Review
- Case Studies
- Videos and Animations

154

© 2011 by Pearson Education, Inc.

19. _____ Polysaccharides
20. _____ Polyunsaturated fatty acid
21. _____ Resting energy
22. _____ Saturated fatty acid
23. _____ Triglycerides
24. _____ Undernutrition
25. _____ Vitamins
26. _____ Water-soluble vitamins

m. A term used to describe tube feedings

n. An acid with more than one double bond

o. The intake of nutrients insufficient to meet daily energy

p. The simplest and most common form of lipids consisting of a glycerol molecule with up to three fatty acids attached

q. Acids categorized as those that cannot be manufactured by the body

r. A measure of fat, muscle, and skeleton

s. A substance the body cannot store so they must be supplied daily and are affected by food processing, storage, and preparation

t. Sugars which may be single molecules

u. The amount of work energy required when a force of 1 Newton (N) moves 1 kilogram of weight 1 meter distance

v. A compound molecule of glucose

w. The rate at which the body metabolizes food to maintain the energy requirements of a person who is awake and at rest

x. Starches that are an insoluble form of carbohydrate that is not sweet because they have branched chains of dozens to hundreds of glucose molecules

y. The amount of heat energy required to raise the temperature of 1 gram of water 15 to 16 degrees Celsius and is the unit used in nutrition

z. Compounds that cannot be manufactured by the body and are needed in small quantities to catalyze metabolic processes

KEY TOPIC REVIEW

27. List six nutrients that are both organic and inorganic substances found in foods.

28. List three major functions of nutrients.

29. List the three chemicals that make up carbohydrates.

30. List the two types of carbohydrates.

31. List the three monosaccharides.

32. List the chemical compounds in protein.

33. List the nine essential amino acids.

34. List the nine nonessential amino acids.

35. List the three types of proteins.

156 CHAPTER 32 / Nutrition

36. List three enzymes secreted by the pancreas.

37. List three activities for protein metabolism.

38. List the water-soluble vitamins.

39. List the fat-soluble vitamins.

40. List 12 things that influence eating habits.

41. List suggestions that may help parents meet the child's nutritional needs and promote effective parent–child interactions.

42. List five things that can contribute to poor nutrition in older adults.

43. List key points of the dietary guidelines.

44. List six keys to good nutrition.

45. List reasons why people become vegetarians.

46. List eight problems associated with inadequate nutrition.

CASE STUDY

47. Jonas, a 34-year-old Orthodox Jewish male, was admitted to the trauma unit following a car accident. His injuries included a fractured pelvis and an open right femur fracture. He was placed in traction and will be on bed rest for up to 6 weeks. He will need to be turned and positioned to prevent decubitus ulcers and will need ROM exercises to maintain strength. His family wants to bring in food to provide foods he likes and to make sure it is kosher.

    1. What are his caloric needs?

    2. What foods need to be eliminated from his diet because of religion?

    3. What can be added to his diet that will help to promote his health?

    4. Will the family be permitted to bring in food? If so, how will calories be calculated?

REVIEW QUESTIONS

48. What is the body's most basic nutrient need?

    a. Vitamins

    b. Minerals

    c. Water

    d. Proteins

49. What helps to satisfy the appetite and helps the digestive tract function effectively to eliminate waste?

    a. Carbohydrates

    b. Proteins

    c. Fats

    d. Fiber

50. What processed food is considered to contain empty calories?

    a. Fiber

    b. Carbohydrates

    c. Proteins

    d. Fats

51. What happens to glucose that cannot be stored as glycogen?

    a. It is converted to fat.

    b. It is removed as a waste product.

    c. It is used as energy.

    d. It breaks down in the liver.

52. What is the combination of two or more vegetables that provide all essential amino acids called?

    a. Complete proteins

    b. Incomplete proteins

    c. Complementary proteins

    d. Vegetarian proteins

53. What in the mouth breaks protein down into smaller units?

    a. Saliva

    b. Bacteria

    c. Teeth

    d. Pepsin

54. How are amino acids absorbed?

    a. Through peristalsis

    b. By active transport

    c. By osmosis

    d. Through filtration

55. Where does the body store the excess amino acids?

    a. Liver

    b. Skeletal system

    c. It cannot store them

    d. Small intestine

56. What is the element that distinguishes proteins from other macronutrients?

    a. Amino acids

    b. Glycogen

    c. Enzymes

    d. Nitrogen

57. What are organic substances that are greasy and insoluble in water but soluble in alcohol or ether?

    a. Proteins

    b. Carbohydrates

    c. Lipids

    d. Fiber

58. What is the simplest and most common form of lipids consisting of a glycerol molecule with up to three fatty acids attached?

    a. Triglyceride

    b. Glyceride

    c. Monoglyceride

    d. Cholesterol

59. What is needed to create bile acids to synthesize steroid hormones?

    a. Glycerides

    b. Triglycerides

    c. Cholesterol

    d. Lipids

60. What is an essential ingredient for brain, nerve, and red blood cells?

    a. Glucose

    b. Cholesterol

    c. Triglycerides

    d. Fats

61. Which vitamins must be supplied daily and are affected by food processing, storage, and preparation?

    a. Water-soluble

    b. Fat-soluble

    c. Calcium

    d. Omega 3's

62. What fat-soluble vitamins can only be stored in limited quantities?

    a. A and E

    b. D and K

    c. B and C

    d. E and K

63. What maintains the basal metabolic rate of the body and provides energy for activities such as running and walking?

    a. Vitamins

    b. Lipids

    c. Fiber

    d. Food

64. What is a major health concern for the young obese adult?

    a. Hypertension

    b. Cardiac problems

    c. Cancer

    d. Arthritis

65. What is the term for obesity that interferes with mobility or breathing?

    a. Overweight

    b. Morbid obesity

    c. Overnutrition

    d. Obesity

66. Where is the most common site for skinfolds measurement?

    a. Waist

    b. Gluteus maximus

    c. Biceps

    d. Triceps

67. What indicates a low serum albumin level?

    a. Low hemoglobin

    b. Prolonged protein depletion

    c. Low transferring

    d. Low hematocrit

CHAPTER 33

Urinary Elimination

KEY TERM REVIEW

Match each term with its appropriate definition.

1. _____ Anuria
2. _____ Credé maneuver
3. _____ Detrusor muscle
4. _____ Dialysis
5. _____ Dysuria
6. _____ Enuresis
7. _____ Habit training
8. _____ Ileal conduit
9. _____ Irrigation
10. _____ Micturition
11. _____ Nephrostomy
12. _____ Neurogenic bladder
13. _____ Nocturia
14. _____ Nocturnal frequency
15. _____ Oliguria
16. _____ Polydipsia
17. _____ Reflux
18. _____ Residual urine
19. _____ Suprapubic catheter
20. _____ Ureterostomy

a. Leakage of urine back toward the kidneys
b. The most common urinary diversion
c. Emptying of the bladder
d. When one or both of the ureters may be brought directly to the side of the abdomen to form small stomas
e. Low urine output, usually less than 500 mL a day or 30 mL an hour for an adult
f. A delayed difficulty in initiating voiding, associated with dysuria
g. A lack of urine production
h. Urine remaining in the bladder following voiding
i. Voiding at frequent intervals of more than four to six times a day
j. Manual pressure on the bladder to promote bladder emptying
k. What may be formed when the bladder is left intact but voiding through the urethra is not possible, due to an obstruction or a neurogenic bladder
l. Muscle tone necessary so the bladder can fill adequately and empty completely

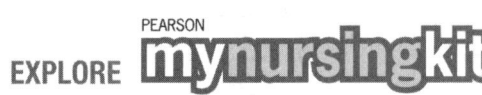

EXPLORE **mynursingkit**

www.mynursingkit.com

MyNursingKit is your one stop for online chapter review materials and resources. Prepare for success with additional NCLEX®-style practice questions, interactive assignments and activities, web links, animations and videos, and more! Register your access code from the front of your textbook at www.mynursingkit.com

Look for these resources:
- NCLEX® Review
- Case Studies
- Videos and Animations

21. _____ Urgency
22. _____ Urinary frequency
23. _____ Urinary hesitancy
24. _____ Urinary retention
25. _____ Vesicostomy
26. _____ Voiding

m. Involuntary urination after control should have been established

n. The flushing or washing out with a specified solution

o. A condition in which the client cannot perceive bladder fullness and is unable to control the urinary sphincters

p. Voiding that is painful or difficult

q. A diversion of urine from the kidney to a stoma

r. A technique by which fluids and molecules pass through a semipermeable membrane according to the rules of osmosis

s. The need for older adults to rise during the night to void

t. Timed voiding and scheduled toiletry to keep clients dry by having them void at regular intervals

u. Emptying of the urinary bladder

v. Voiding two or more times at night

w. A catheter inserted surgically through the abdominal wall above the symphysis pubis into the urinary bladder

x. Can follow excessive fluid intake or may be associated with diseases such as diabetes mellitus, diabetes insipidus, and chronic nephritis

y. When emptying of the bladder is impaired, urine accumulates, and the bladder becomes overdistended

z. A strong sudden desire to void

KEY TOPIC REVIEW

27. List three urinary habits.

28. List three things that affect personal habits regarding urination.

29. List five things that effective urinary elimination depends on.

30. List five things that glomerular filtrate is made up of.

31. List the four layers that make up the wall of the bladder.

32. List problems caused for older adults by altering normal fluid intake and output.

33. List common complaints related to the bladder.

34. List conditions that help stimulate the micturition reflex.

35. List three diseases that might be associated with polydipsia.

36. List five things that polyuria can cause.

37. List the two forms of dialysis.

38. List manifestations of underlying conditions such as a urinary tract infection.

162 CHAPTER 33 / Urinary Elimination

39. List manifestations or primary problems affecting urinary elimination.

40. List eight common causes of incontinence.

41. List nine factors that can contribute to acute or reversible incontinence.

42. List five different types of chronic incontinence, each having a different etiology.

43. List inorganic solutes found in urine.

44. List three tests related to urinary functions.

45. List overall goals for clients with urinary elimination problems.

CASE STUDY

46. Maude, an 86-year-old female, was transferred from the hospital following bladder surgery to a long-term care facility. She is a widow with no relatives to help her. Maude has had cancerous polyps in the bladder that have been removed several times, but they finally had to remove the bladder and place a ureterostomy for urinary drainage. Due to her age and arthritic hands, she is unable to care for her appliance. She will need constant care and monitoring for problems such as leakage and infections.

    1. Since she is 86, will body image be a problem for her?

    2. How often will the bag be replaced?

    3. Is there a problem with infections with a ureterostomy?

    4. Who will provide the necessary care for the appliance?

REVIEW QUESTIONS

47. What are the functional units of the kidneys?

    a. Ureters

    b. Nephrons

    c. Glomerulus

    d. Bowman's capsule

48. Where is most of the water and electrolytes reabsorbed?

    a. Proximal convoluted tubule

    b. Loop of Henle

    c. Bowman's capsule

    d. Distal convoluted tubule

49. What is a hollow, muscular organ that serves as a reservoir for urine and as the organ of excretion?

    a. Ureters

    b. Kidneys

    c. Urethra

    d. Bladder

50. What is the involuntary passing of urine during sleep?

    a. Enuresis

    b. Nocturnal enuresis

    c. Secondary enuresis

    d. Oliguria

51. What places the older adult at higher risk for toxicity from medications if excretion rates are longer?

    a. Liver disease

    b. Arteriosclerosis

    c. Kidney disease

    d. Peripheral vascular disease

52. What predisposes the older adult to bladder infections?

    a. Retention of residual urine

    b. Nocturnal frequency

    c. Holding the urine too long

    d. Enuresis

53. What behavior can increase the risk of urinary tract infections?

    a. Muscle tension

    b. Ignoring the urge to void

    c. Anxiety

    d. Voiding by time factors

54. What can increase fluid output by inhibiting the production of antidiuretic hormone?

    a. Water

    b. Soda

    c. Juice

    d. Alcohol

55. What food can cause urine to turn red?

    a. Carotene

    b. Apples

    c. Strawberries

    d. Beets

56. What group of medications can increase urine formation by preventing the reabsorption of water and electrolytes from the tubules of the kidney into the bloodstream?

    a. Antibiotics

    b. Hypertensives

    c. Diuretics

    d. Antipsychotics

© 2011 by Pearson Education, Inc.

CHAPTER 33 / Urinary Elimination

57. What contributes to the ability to store and empty urine?

    a. Bladder

    b. Urethra

    c. Pelvic muscle tone

    d. Detrusor muscle

58. What is a sensitive indicator of renal function?

    a. Creatinine

    b. Urea

    c. Glomerular filtration rate

    d. BUN

59. What is nursing care of the client with an indwelling catheter directed toward?

    a. Preventing infection

    b. Maintaining output

    c. Emptying catheter

    d. Recording I & O

60. What can be formed when the bladder is left intact but voiding through the urethra is not possible?

    a. Ureterostomy

    b. Nephrostomy

    c. Vesicostomy

    d. Ileal loop

61. What are clients who must wear a urine collection appliance at risk for?

    a. Infection

    b. Excoriation

    c. Impaired skin integrity

    d. Inflammation

62. What problems do clients with urinary diversions experience?

    a. Lifestyles

    b. Body image

    c. Coping

    d. Stress

CHAPTER 34

FECAL ELIMINATION

KEY TERM REVIEW

Match each term with its appropriate definition.

1. _____ Bowel incontinence
2. _____ Carminatives
3. _____ Cathartics
4. _____ Colostomy
5. _____ Constipation
6. _____ Defecation
7. _____ Diarrhea
8. _____ Enema
9. _____ Fecal impaction
10. _____ Feces
11. _____ Flatulence
12. _____ Flatus
13. _____ Gastrocolic reflux
14. _____ Gastrostomy
15. _____ Hemorrhoids
16. _____ Ileostomy
17. _____ Jejunostomy
18. _____ Laxatives
19. _____ Mass peristalsis
20. _____ Meconium

a. Excreted waste products

b. Distended veins within the rectum occurring due to repeated pressure when excreting feces

c. Laxatives given to soften the feces by releasing gas such as carbon dioxide to distend the rectum, or by stimulating nerve endings in the rectal mucosa

d. The loss of voluntary ability to control fecal and gaseous discharges through the anal sphincter

e. The first fecal material passed by a newborn, normally 24 hours after birth

f. Gas forming in the large intestine, usually forming 7 to 10 L every 24 hours

g. Increased peristalsis of the colon after food has entered the stomach

h. The opening created in the abdominal wall, generally red in color and moist

i. Herbal oils known to act as agents that help expel gas from the stomach and intestines

j. An opening into the small bowel which produces liquid fecal draining

k. Drugs used to induce defecation

l. A condition defined as having fewer than three bowel movements per week

EXPLORE mynursingkit

www.mynursingkit.com

MyNursingKit is your one stop for online chapter review materials and resources. Prepare for success with additional NCLEX®-style practice questions, interactive assignments and activities, web links, animations and videos, and more! Register your access code from the front of your textbook at www.mynursingkit.com

Look for these resources:
- NCLEX® Review
- Case Studies
- Videos and Animations

21. _____ Ostomy
22. _____ Peristalsis
23. _____ Stoma
24. _____ Suppositories

m. An opening for the gastrointestinal, urinary, or respiratory tract, onto the skin

n. An opening into the large bowel to divert and drain fecal material

o. Defecation when the urge is recognized for regular bowel elimination

p. Expulsion of feces from the anus and rectum

q. An opening through the abdominal wall into the stomach

r. The passage of liquid feces and an increased frequency of defecation

s. The presence of excessive flatus in the intestines which leads to stretching and inflation of the intestines (intestinal distention)

t. Medication that stimulates bowel activity and assists fecal elimination

u. A solution introduced into the rectum and large intestine to increase peristalsis for the excretion of feces and flatulence

v. An opening through the abdominal wall into the jejunum

w. A mass or collection of hardened feces in the folds of the rectum, which resulted from prolonged retention and accumulation of fecal material

x. Activity stimulating the facilitating of movement of chyme along the colon

KEY TOPIC REVIEW

25. List the seven parts of the colon.

26. List the colon's main functions.

27. List gases contained in flatus.

28. List six circumstances of diet that affect defecation patterns.

29. List three essential preventive measures for constipation.

30. List eight foods that may influence bowel elimination.

31. List reasons for weak abdominal and pelvic muscles.

32. List four common problems that are related to fecal elimination.

33. List 12 causes and factors that contribute to constipation.

34. List serious problems that the Valsalva maneuver can present.

35. List eight of the major causes of diarrhea and the physiologic responses of the body.

36. List two types of bowel incontinence.

37. List three primary sources of flatus.

38. List classifications of bowel diversion ostomies.

39. List types of stoma construction.

40. List six things the nurse needs to observe with the client's stool.

41. List the major goals for clients with fecal elimination problems.

42. List ways the nurse can help clients achieve regular defecation.

43. List the most common categories of medications affecting fecal elimination.

44. List problems that contraindicate the use of laxatives.

CASE STUDY

45. Sandy, a 33-year-old female, was suffering from a rectal-vaginal fistula that developed during the birth of her daughter. She finally decided to have it repaired and was told it would require a temporary colostomy needed to allow the area to heal. Sandy did not like the idea of caring for a colostomy, but after several years of dealing with fecal drainage from the vaginal area she felt she could handle it and opted for the surgery. After going through all the pre-op she was cleared for the procedure. The ostomy nurse did some preliminary teaching and marked the best spot for the doctor to place the colostomy. The next day she was operated on. All went well except the tissue in the vaginal area was friable and the surgeon had problems finding healthy tissue to repair the opening. He did the best he could and sent the client to the recovery room. When she woke up the surgeon informed her that the colostomy would have to be permanent because of the poor tissue quality. Sandy was very upset and wished she had left it the way it was.

    1. What teaching will she need to maintain the colostomy?
    2. Would she have been better off not having the surgery?
    3. Why was the tissue friable?
    4. Would a support group be beneficial for Sandy to help her get through this?

REVIEW QUESTIONS

46. What regulates the flow of chyme into the large intestine and prevents backflow into the ileum?

    a. Ileocecal valve

    b. Internal sphincter

    c. External sphincter

    d. Cardiac sphincter

47. How does the feces move into the sigmoid colon and the rectum?

    a. Defecation

    b. Bowel movement

    c. Peristaltic waves

    d. Rugae

48. What is a result if defecation is consciously inhibited by contracting the external sphincter muscle?

    a. Diarrhea

    b. Constipation

    c. Incontinence

    d. Flatus

49. What bacterium affects the color of feces?

    a. Escherichia coli

    b. Pseudomonas

    c. Streptococci

    d. Clostridium difficile

50. What is the most common bowel-management problem in the older adult population?

    a. Flatus

    b. Diarrhea

    c. Constipation

    d. Incontinence

51. When is the gastrocolic reflex the strongest?

    a. Early in the morning

    b. In the evening

    c. 5 to 15 minutes after meals

    d. In the afternoon

52. What inhibits natural defecation reflexes and is thought to cause rather than cure constipation?

    a. Valsalva maneuver

    b. Prunes

    c. Laxatives

    d. Suppositories

53. What can be recognized by the passage of liquid fecal seepage and no normal stool?

    a. Diarrhea

    b. Constipation

    c. Flatulence

    d. Fecal impaction

54. What results from rapid movement of fecal contents through the large intestine?

    a. Constipation

    b. Diarrhea

    c. Fecal impaction

    d. Normal defecation

55. What is a protective flushing mechanism?

    a. Constipation

    b. Fecal impaction

    c. Defecation

    d. Diarrhea

56. What influences the character and management of the fecal drainage in an ostomy?

    a. Location

    b. Foods ingested

    c. Amount of fluids

    d. Activities

57. Which colostomy produces increasingly solid fecal drainage?

    a. Ascending

    b. Descending

    c. Transverse

    d. Ileostomy

58. What type of colostomy has a loop of bowel brought out onto the abdominal wall and supported by a plastic bridge, or a piece of rubber tubing?

    a. Loop

    b. Single

    c. Double-barreled

    d. Divided

59. What weakens the bowel's natural responses to fecal distention, resulting in chronic constipation?

    a. Fiber

    b. Laxatives

    c. Enemas

    d. Antacids

60. What solution exerts a lower osmotic pressure than the surrounding interstitial fluid, causing water to move from the colon into the interstitial space?

    a. Hypotonic

    b. Hypertonic

    c. Isotonic

    d. Carminative enema

61. What can cause an excessive vagal response resulting in cardiac arrhythmia?

    a. Enemas

    b. Suppositories

    c. Rectal stimulation

    d. Disimpaction

CHAPTER 35

OXYGENATION AND CIRCULATION

KEY TERM REVIEW

Match each term with its appropriate definition.

1. _____ Adventitious breath sounds
2. _____ Apnea
3. _____ Atelectasis
4. _____ Atherosclerosis
5. _____ Biot's (cluster) respiration
6. _____ Bradypnea
7. _____ Cheyne-Stokes respirations
8. _____ Cyanosis
9. _____ Dyspnea
10. _____ Emphysema
11. _____ Eupnea
12. _____ Expectorate
13. _____ Hemothorax
14. _____ Hypercapnia
15. _____ Hyperinflation
16. _____ Intrapleural pressure
17. _____ Ischemia
18. _____ Kussmaul's breathing

a. Spit out
b. The compound of oxygen and hemoglobin
c. An abnormally slow respiratory rate
d. Enzyme that is released into the blood during a myocardial infarction (MI)
e. Normal respiration which is quiet, rhythmic, and effortless
f. Drainage by gravity of secretions from various lung segments
g. Abnormal breath sounds
h. A lipoprotein produced by specialized alveolar cells, acts like a detergent, reducing the surface tension of alveolar fluid
i. The cessation of breathing
j. Heart attack
k. A collapse of a portion of the lung
l. A harsh high-pitched sound which may be heard during inspiration
m. The buildup of fatty plaque in the arteries
n. Air collected in the pleural space

19. _____ Lung recoil
20. _____ Myocardial infarction
21. _____ Oxyhemoglobin
22. _____ Pneumothorax
23. _____ Postural drainage
24. _____ Stridor
25. _____ Surfactant
26. _____ Troponin

o. Shallow breaths interrupted by apnea

p. Marked rhythmic waxing and waning of respirations from deep to very shallow breathing

q. The continual tendency of the lungs to collapse away from the chest wall

r. The giving of a client breaths that are 1 to 1.5 times the tidal volume set on the ventilator through the ventilation circuit or via a manual resuscitation bag

s. Blood or fluid in the pleural space placing pressure on lung tissue and interfering with lung expansion

t. A condition in which carbon dioxide often accumulates in the blood

u. Bluish discoloration of the skin, nail beds, and mucous membranes due to reduced hemoglobin oxygen saturation

v. Difficult or uncomfortable breathing

w. Pressure in the cavity surrounding the lungs, slightly negative in relation to atmospheric pressure

x. A type of hyperventilation that accompanies metabolic acidosis by which the body attempts to compensate by blowing off carbon dioxide through deep and rapid breathing

y. The lack of blood supply due to obstructed circulation

z. A chronic lung ailment in which oxygen concentrations, not carbon dioxide concentrations, play a major role in regulating respiration

KEY TOPIC REVIEW

27. List the three components involved in the process of respiration.

28. List factors needed for adequate ventilation.

29. List factors that affect the rate of oxygen transport from the lungs to the tissues.

30. List the three blood gases that can trigger chemoreceptors.

31. List the accessory muscles of respiration.

32. List factors that influence oxygenation.

33. List changes that compromise the respiratory system.

34. List four things in the environment that affect oxygenation.

35. List symptoms that healthy people experience when exposed to air pollution.

36. List medications that can decrease the rate and depth of respirations.

37. List two things epinephrine causes.

38. List three major alterations in respirations.

39. List the parts of respiration.

40. List the four types of breathing.

41. List what breathing pattern refers to.

42. List six things a nurse should glean from a client's history relevant to oxygenation status.

43. List the four physical examination techniques.

44. List various diagnostic tests to assess respiratory status, function, and oxygenation.

45. List the overall outcomes/goals for a client with oxygenation problems.

46. List nine examples of nursing interventions to facilitate pulmonary ventilation.

47. List interventions that the nurse would use to maintain normal respirations of clients.

48. List seven adverse effects of codeine when added to cough syrups.

CASE STUDY

49. Joseph, a 53-year-old male, has been a two-pack-a-day smoker for over 30 years. He came to the emergency department with shortness of breath and a productive cough that he has had for at least 10 years, but it has gotten worse and he is occasionally coughing up blood. He does not have a regular doctor and has not had a physical exam for more than 15 years. He works in a steel mill and is exposed to high heat and fumes from the molten metals. His vital signs are 102, 90, 24, 116/74, and oxygen saturation of 85%. An IV was started and an ECG was done showing premature ventricular contractions (PVCs).

    1. What is the cause of the distress?

    2. What are some things the nurse needs to teach the client to improve his health status?

    3. How much oxygen will he need to bring him to a satisfactory level?

    4. Is he sick enough to be admitted or will he be sent home with medications?

REVIEW QUESTIONS

50. What mechanisms work to keep airways open and clear in order for gas exchange to occur?

    a. Ciliary action and the cough reflex

    b. The medulla and pons

    c. Expansion and recoil

    d. Visceral pleura and parietal pleura

51. What is the movement of gases or other particles from an area of greater pressure or concentration to an area of lower pressure or concentration?

    a. Osmosis

    b. Diffusion

    c. Transport

    d. Respiration

52. What is needed for respiratory regulation to maintain the correct concentrations of oxygen, carbon dioxide, and hydrogen ions in body fluids?

    a. PO_2 and PCO_2

    b. Arterial blood gases

    c. Both neural and chemical controls

    d. C-PAP

53. What lipoprotein is needed for lung expansion?

    a. Glycogen

    b. Glucose

    c. Protease

    d. Surfactant

54. What increases the rate and depth of respirations and the supply of oxygen in the body?

    a. Exercise

    b. Sleep

    c. Rest

    d. Smoking

55. What is an abnormally slow respiratory rate, which may be seen in clients who have taken drugs such as morphine, who have metabolic alkalosis, or who have increased intracranial pressure?

    a. Apnea

    b. Tachypnea

    c. Bradypnea

    d. Eupnea

56. What is an increased movement of air into and out of the lungs called?

    a. Kussmaul's breathing

    b. Hypoventilation

    c. Hyperventilation

    d. Tachypnea

57. What cannot be directly observed or measured but is reported by the client?

    a. Dyspnea

    b. Orthopnea

    c. Eupnea

    d. Tachypnea

CHAPTER 35 / Oxygenation and Circulation

58. What do clients with emphysema frequently develop?

    a. Bronchitis

    b. COPD

    c. Barrel chest

    d. Flail chest

59. What do decongestants contain that can increase heart rate and respiratory rate, and result in insomnia due to its stimulant effects?

    a. Codeine

    b. Pseudoephedrine

    c. Epinephrine

    d. Leukotrienes

60. How do the upper lobes of the lungs drain?

    a. By gravity

    b. By coughing

    c. By deep breathing

    d. By suctioning

61. What happens when free-flowing oxygen is ignited?

    a. Nothing.

    b. It will have an odor.

    c. It will burn.

    d. It will explode.

62. How is humidity provided to a client with a tracheostomy?

    a. Via face mask

    b. Via nasal cannula

    c. By mist collar

    d. By a rebreather

63. Which of the following devices can attach to the chest tube and has a one-way valve and a small built-in collection chamber?

    a. Pneumostat

    b. Heimlich valve

    c. Suction catheter

    d. Ventilator

64. What is the major transport system of the body, bringing oxygen and nutrients to the cells and removing wastes for disposal?

    a. Respiratory system

    b. Urinary system

    c. Cardiovascular system

    d. Vascular system

65. What supplies the heart muscle with oxygen or nourishment from the blood?

    a. Coronary arteries

    b. Atrials

    c. Ventricles

    d. Carotid arteries

66. What can generate an electrical impulse and contraction independently of the nervous system?

    a. The brain

    b. The spinal cord

    c. Skeletal muscle

    d. Cardiac muscle

67. What serves as the transport medium within the cardiovascular system, bringing oxygen and nutrients from the environment to the cells?

    a. Plasma

    b. Electrolytes

    c. Blood

    d. Carbon dioxide

68. What is known as the silent killer because of its lack of symptoms and is a major risk factor for sudden cardiac death in middle adulthood?

    a. Hypotension

    b. Hypertension

    c. Arteriosclerosis

    d. Atherosclerosis

69. What is an amino acid that has been shown to be increased in many people with atherosclerosis?

    a. Valine

    b. Homocysteine

    c. Glycine

    d. Alanine

CHAPTER 36

FLUID, ELECTROLYTE, AND ACID–BASE BALANCE

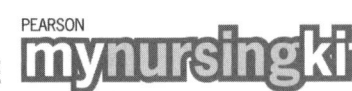

KEY TERM REVIEW

Match each term with its appropriate definition.

1. _____ Alkalosis
2. _____ Anions
3. _____ Cations
4. _____ Colloidal osmotic pressure
5. _____ Crystalloids
6. _____ Diffusion
7. _____ Electrolytes
8. _____ Filtration
9. _____ Fluid volume deficit
10. _____ Hematocrit
11. _____ Hydrostatic pressure
12. _____ Hyperkalemia
13. _____ Hyperphosphatemia
14. _____ Insensible fluid loss
15. _____ Interstitial fluid
16. _____ Intravascular fluid
17. _____ Isotonic
18. _____ Metabolic alkalosis
19. _____ Obligatory losses
20. _____ Osmolality

a. The continual intermingling of molecules in liquids, gases, or solids brought about by the random movement of their molecules

b. A potassium excess or a serum potassium level greater than 5.0 mEq/L

c. Charged particles capable of conducting electricity

d. Fluids which include cerebrospinal, pericardial, pancreatic, pleural, intraocular, biliary, peritoneal, and synovial

e. Normal saline solution, 0.9% sodium chloride

f. Ions that carry a negative charge such as chloride, bicarbonate, phosphate, and sulfate

g. A small depression or pit after finger pressure is applied to a swollen area

h. Salts that dissolve readily into true solutions

i. A loss occurring through the skin and lungs which is usually not noticeable and cannot be measured

j. Ions that carry a positive charge, such as sodium, potassium, calcium, and magnesium

k. Cell membranes which allow solutes to move across them with ease

EXPLORE mynursingkit

www.mynursingkit.com

MyNursingKit is your one stop for online chapter review materials and resources. Prepare for success with additional NCLEX®-style practice questions, interactive assignments and activities, web links, animations and videos, and more! Register your access code from the front of your textbook at www.mynursingkit.com

Look for these resources:
- NCLEX® Review
- Case Studies
- Videos and Animations

21. _____ Pitting edema
22. _____ Renin angiotensin-aldosterone system
23. _____ Respiratory acidosis
24. _____ Selectively permeable
25. _____ Solutes
26. _____ Transcellular fluids

l. Plasma proteins exerting an osmotic draw, pulling water from the interstitial space into the vascular compartment

m. The concentration of solutes in body fluids, reported as milliosmols per kilogram (mOsm/kg)

n. A process whereby fluid and solutes move together across a membrane from one compartment to another

o. Hypoventilation and carbon dioxide retention cause carbonic acid levels to increase and the pH level to fall below 7.35

p. The occurrence when the body loses both water and electrolytes from the ECF (extracellular fluid) in similar proportions

q. A system initiated by specialized receptors in the juxtaglomerular cells of the kidney nephrons responding to changes in renal perfusion

r. Pressure exerted by a fluid within a closed system on the walls of a container in which it is contained

s. Fluid losses required to maintain normal body functions

t. The measure of volume (percentage) of whole blood that is composed of RBCs

u. Plasma which accounts for approximately 20% of the ECF found within the vascular system

v. Defined in adults as a total serum phosphate level greater than 4.5 mg/dL, which occurs when phosphate shifts out of the cells into extracellular fluids

w. A fluid surrounding the cells which accounts for approximately 75% of the extracellular fluid

x. Substances dissolved in liquid

y. A state characterized by a decrease in the hydrogen ion concentration of arterial blood below the normal level, when the pH rises

z. A condition when the amount of bicarbonate in the body exceeds the normal 20-to-1 ratio

KEY TOPIC REVIEW

27. List eight functions of water.

28. List the body's two major fluid compartments.

29. List the solutes contained in the intracellular fluid.

30. List chemicals found in extracellular and intracellular fluids.

31. List three things that affect total body water.

32. List eight examples of transcellular fluid.

33. List the principal electrolytes in extracellular fluid.

34. List causes for fluid and electrolyte imbalances.

35. List the methods by which electrolytes and other solutes move.

36. List seven solutes in the body.

37. List the primary contributors to the osmolality of intracellular fluid.

38. List the four routes of fluid output.

39. List the factors that can affect the body's ability to maintain fluid, electrolyte, and acid–base balance.

40. List three things that can cause significant fluid loss.

41. List five body systems that contribute to the regulation of homeostasis.

42. List factors that affect the production and release of ADH.

43. List things electrolytes are important for.

44. List vital actions performed by calcium.

45. List eight sources of magnesium.

46. List things that need to be assessed when the client has a subclavian central venous catheter.

CASE STUDY

47. Julia, a 26-year-old female, called her personal physician after spending three days at home with nausea, vomiting, and diarrhea. On the day she got sick, she had eaten at a new fish restaurant. She has not been able to eat or drink anything that stays down and is getting worried. She feels weak and has lost 6 pounds. She sleeps when she is not in the bathroom, but her heart feels funny and she is dizzy when she stands up. She lives alone so no one is around to help her out and she needs to get back to work or she could lose her job.

    1. What is her problem?

    2. What kind of treatment will she need?

    3. What is causing the heart to feel funny?

    4. What are some tests that need to be done?

REVIEW QUESTIONS

48. What age group has the highest proportion of water, accounting for 70% to 80% of their body weight?

    a. Teens

    b. Adults

    c. Infants

    d. Children

49. What is the transport system that carries nutrients to and waste products from the cells?

    a. Intracellular fluid

    b. Extracellular fluid

    c. Intravascular fluid

    d. Interstitial fluid

50. What is a protein-rich fluid containing a large amount of albumin?

    a. Plasma

    b. Blood

    c. Extracellular fluid

    d. Intracellular fluid

51. What are the primary cations present in ICF?

    a. Sodium and chloride

    b. Potassium and sodium

    c. Phosphate and sulfate

    d. Potassium and magnesium

52. What is an important mechanism for maintaining homeostasis and fluid balance?

    a. Diffusion

    b. Osmosis

    c. Filtration

    d. Active transport

53. What two major systems work on a continuous basis to help regulate the acid–base balance in the body?

    a. Lungs and kidneys

    b. Liver and pancreas

    c. Heart and kidneys

    d. Heart and lungs

54. Which hormone is synthesized in the anterior portion of the hypothalamus and acts on the collecting ducts of the nephrons?

    a. Insulin

    b. Angiotensin

    c. Antidiuretic hormone

    d. Aldosterone

55. Which of the following is a vital electrolyte for skeletal, cardiac, and smooth muscle activity?

    a. Sodium

    b. Calcium

    c. Potassium

    d. Chloride

56. What is the richest source of calcium?

    a. Bananas

    b. Salmon

    c. Milk

    d. Cheese

57. What is a measure of the metabolic component of acid–base balance?

    a. Base excess

    b. $PaCO_2$

    c. Bicarbonate HCO_3

    d. PaO_2

58. Which solution is often used to restore vascular volume?

    a. Hypotonic

    b. Hypertonic

    c. Isotonic

    d. Nutrient

59. What catheters are frequently used for long-term intravenous access when the client will be managing IV therapy at home?

    a. Central venous

    b. PICC

    c. Jugular

    d. Peripheral

60. Which age groups are especially at risk for complications of fluid overload with rapid IV infusion?

    a. Older adults and pediatric clients

    b. Teens and infants

    c. Geriatrics and middle-aged adults

    d. Adults and pediatric clients

61. What should always be used when giving a blood transfusion?

    a. Lactated Ringer's

    b. $D_{10}W$

    c. D_5W

    d. Normal saline

62. How is fluid intake regulated?

    a. By checking skin turgor

    b. By drinking 8 glasses of water a day

    c. By thirst

    d. By hunger

Answer Key

Chapter 1

1. f 2. h 3. c 4. b 5. j 6. k
7. a 8. d 9. i 10. e 11. g
12. American Nurses Association, National League for Nursing, International Council of Nurses, National Student Nurses' Association
13. Dorothea Orem, Betty Neuman, Hildegard Peplau, Madeleine Leininger, Jean Watson
14. requirement of prolonged, specialized training to acquire a body of knowledge pertinent to the role to be performed; an orientation of the individual toward service, either to a community or to an organization; ongoing research; a code of ethics; autonomy; a professional organization
15. novice, advanced beginner, competent, proficient, expert
16. caring; an art; a science; client-centered; holistic; adaptive; concerned with health promotion, maintenance, and restoration; and a helping profession
17. Lillian Wald and Mary Brewster
18. promoting health and wellness, preventing illness, restoring health, caring for the dying
19. provide immunizations, prenatal and infant care, and prevention of STIs
20. hospital diploma, associate degree, baccalaureate degree, master's degree, doctoral degree
21. homes, hospitals, and extended care facilities
22. negligence, malpractice, invasion of privacy, and assault or battery
23. (1) Nurses need to have a variety of skills. With her interests and skills she may work well as a nurse manager or in a clinic or physician's office. (2) There are opportunities in management or education. (3) Computers are being used in all facilities, often even in a client's room. Laptops are used for visiting nurses. (4) Going back to school for an MSN could open the doors as a nurse educator or even to work as a nurse practitioner. Continued education is always a plus.
24. c. *Rationale:* We still celebrate Florence Nightingale's birthday every year, and many programs use the lamp during the graduation ceremony.
25. b. *Rationale:* Mary Mahoney is the only African American nurse listed.
26. b. *Rationale:* Margaret Sanger was imprisoned for opening a birth control information clinic. Her experience with the large number of unwanted pregnancies among the working poor influenced her to address this problem.
27. c. *Rationale:* Watson believed the practice of caring is central to nursing.
28. a. *Rationale:* Research in any profession will help to advance a profession. Nursing needs to continue to grow and become a profession that governs itself.
29. c. *Rationale:* Although some of the other answers have been used to identify nursing in a loose context, c is the most complete.
30. b. *Rationale:* Those listed were healers and precursors to nurses. Traditional healers, particularly midwives, were favored targets of the medieval witch hunts.
31. a. *Rationale:* Deaconesses set up some of the first hospitals.
32. c. *Rationale:* The nurse practice acts guide nurses to what they can legally do in their state.
33. d. *Rationale:* Clara Barton organized nursing services and started the Red Cross.
34. a. *Rationale:* She participated in protest movements for women's rights that resulted in the 1920 passage of the 19th Amendment to the U.S. Constitution, which granted women the right to vote.
35. b. *Rationale:* All those answers can provide health information but the Internet is the fastest growing and easily accessible. The concern is that the information may not be accurate.
36. c. *Rationale:* Nursing schools teach all the answers but they need to change with the times and teach the current trends to remain on the cutting edge of nursing.
37. d. *Rationale:* The state board of nursing found in each state oversees and provides guidance to the profession.

Chapter 2

1. x 2. g 3. s 4. h 5. r 6. u
7. f 8. v 9. w 10. v 11. a 12. k
13. p 14. i 15. c 16. q 17. o 18. j
19. n 20. l 21. e 22. d 23. t 24. b

25. collaboration, communication, compromise
26. chemically dependent on drugs or alcohol, mental illness
27. the nurse's job description, education, expertise, individual institutional policies and procedures
28. public law, private or civil law
29. negligence, malpractice, invasion of privacy, assault or battery
30. breach of confidentiality, fraud, refusing care to clients
31. the consent must be voluntary, the client must be capable and literate, the client must be competent
32. U.S. Constitution, statutes, administrative agencies, and decisions of the courts known as common law
33. complaint, answer, discovery, trial, verdict
34. licensure, certification, and accreditation
35. maternal–child health, pediatrics, mental health, gerontology, or critical care nursing
36. nurse's job description, education, and expertise as well as individual institutional policies and procedures
37. duty, breach of duty, foreseeability, causation, harm or injury
38. medication errors, falls, ignoring a client's complaint, failure to answer a call bell, and incorrectly identifying clients
39. (1) Medication errors are the leading cause of death, and clients can sue the facility and the nurse. The "deep pockets" would be the facility first, then the nurse. (2) Since the nurse works for the hospital, the hospital is responsible for all errors. (3) Policies should be in place to provide an updated reporting system between the units so both nurses are kept informed as well as a charting system that charts once the medication has been dispensed. (4) If this was a mistake she will not lose her license, but it will go on her record and she may be sent for classes to prevent it from happening again. Accountability is a primary concept in the practice of nursing!
40. d. *Rationale:* All the answers except d might create more problems for the facility and the nurse. The facility's lawyer would be the only person who could give advice to nurses being deposed.
41. a. *Rationale:* Refusing to care for a client is illegal and unethical. All clients should be treated equally.
42. d. *Rationale:* The client and her insurance company would be responsible. If the admitting nurse followed all facility policies, the nurse and the facility could not be held accountable.
43. a. *Rationale:* It is implied when a client is admitted that the client will receive the care needed to improve his or her health. Expressed consent would be a verbal contract. Informed consent is usually when a physician explains surgery or a procedure to the client and the client agrees to have it done regardless of the risks. Expected care could be another way to state the obvious, but legally implied is the correct term.
44. a. *Rationale:* Each state sets up nurse practice acts to establish what nurses can and cannot do. These acts do protect the client from harm. Nurses, unless practitioners, can only write orders they receive verbally from a physician. Physicians are responsible for the orders they write, but ultimately the nurse that carries out the order will be responsible if it was unsafe.
45. b. *Rationale:* Employers are responsible for selecting, orienting, and educating employees to the policies of the facility. Nurses are responsible for their actions and are not above the law. They also are not superior to other employees. Medical professionals and UAPs should work as a team.
46. a. *Rationale:* Nurses should always carry a liability policy just for extra protection, but they should not offer diagnoses or care to others that is not authorized.
47. c. *Rationale:* That is the only correct answer.
48. d. *Rationale:* Although all the terms have a similar meaning, the legal term used is whistle-blower.
49. b. *Rationale:* The Good Samaritan act helps to protect nurses and other medical professionals from lawsuits if they perform care in the same way that others would do.
50. d. *Rationale:* Documentation is one of the most important aspects of care. You can be the best nurse in the world and always do things correctly, but if it is not documented there is no proof it was done.
51. b. *Rationale:* Euthanasia is also called mercy killing. We do not have a law that permits clients' lives to be ended through an illegal act of murder. This is a criminal act, but that is not the best answer to the question.
52. c. *Rationale:* The department of health is responsible for the SBON. The other answers are agencies that work for the professionalism of nursing.

Chapter 3

1. b   2. i   3. c   4. k   5. a   6. n
7. m   8. j   9. h   10. d   11. o   12. g
13. l   14. e   15. f
16. primary prevention (health promotion and illness prevention), secondary prevention (diagnosis and treatment), tertiary prevention (rehabilitation, restoration, and palliative care)
17. increase quality and years of healthy life, eliminate health disparities
18. cost of replacing equipment and technology, inflation, increasing older population, increased prescription costs, increase in uninsured, more frequent interaction with health care providers
19. increasing number of older adults, advances in knowledge and technology, economics, increased emphasis on women's health, uneven distribution of health services, access to health care, health care of the homeless and poor, HIPAA, and demographic changes
20. accessibility of health care services, health promotion and disease prevention, and steps to consider how health care costs can be reduced

21. official or public agencies, voluntary or private not-for-profit agencies, private proprietary agencies, and institution-based agencies
22. advocate, caregiver, educator, and case manager
23. plans, implements, and supervises care; teaches clients and their families self-care; and mobilizes the resources of hospitals, primary care providers, and community agencies
24. preventive health education, annual employee health screening for tuberculosis, maintaining immunization information, screening for health problems such as hypertension and obesity, providing care for employees following injury, and offering counseling services
25. inpatient beds, emergency services, diagnostic facilities, ambulatory surgery centers, pharmacy services, intensive and coronary care services, and multiple outpatient services provided by clinics
26. meals, laundry services, nursing care, transportation, and social activities
27. nurses, alternative health care providers, case managers, dentists, dietitians, nutritionists, occupational therapists, paramedical technologists, pharmacists, physical therapists, physicians, physician assistants, spiritual support personnel, podiatrists, respiratory therapists, social workers, unlicensed assistive personnel
28. infectious diseases (e.g., tuberculosis, AIDS), problems with substance abuse, rape, violence, and chronic diseases
29. (1) Social services and financial services can obtain an emergency Medicaid card for clients without insurance. (2) Loans are a possibility, but usually payments can be made to the facility without interest. (3) Nurses as a rule should not get involved in financial issues with their clients. (4) Hospitals provide care and often forgo the payment if it would be a hardship on the client. This is part of community service.
30. c. *Rationale*: *Healthy People 2010* was established to improve the health of the country. The other answers are also issues to be resolved, especially with health care reform.
31. c. *Rationale:* That is the only correct answer. Although nurses do take over for families, usually the families are still there.
32. c. *Rationale:* The population over age 85 is projected to grow the fastest. With new medical procedures and medicines, life expectancy is getting longer.
33. d. *Rationale:* Most people think that a higher rate of the elderly end up in a long-term care facility, but in fact it is only about 5%.
34. d. *Rationale:* These answers all are correct to a degree and all problems caused by low income and lack of medical insurance.
35. a. *Rationale:* Disability is part of Social Security and requires a minimum number of credit years to qualify.
36. d. *Rationale:* Most private insurance is purchased through an organization, most often an employer.
37. b. *Rationale:* Health maintenance organizations were set up to control health issues through preventive measures.
38. b. *Rationale:* Nurses should always get involved with their professional organizations to help promote the profession and set a course for the next generation of nurses.
39. d. *Rationale:* Community-based health care looks out for local industry and proposed changes in the area that could affect the health of the community.
40. d. *Rationale:* With new technology, we can set up cameras and equipment that will send messages back to an office so clients can be monitored but stay in their own homes.
41. c. *Rationale:* Critical pathways establish guidelines to follow a pattern of care and issues during the surgical period. The other answers are nursing theories.

Chapter 4

1. j 2. k 3. h 4. d 5. e 6. c
7. a 8. r 9. q 10. i 11. t 12. p
13. l 14. b 15. s 16. x 17. v 18. m
19. w 20. u 21. o 22. g 23. f 24. n
25. thoughts, communications, actions, customs, beliefs, values, and institutions of racial, ethnic, religious, or social groups
26. providing nutrition and shelter, caring for and educating children, dividing labor, developing social organization, controlling disease, and maintaining health
27. occupational, societal, and ethnic groups
28. race, gender, sexual orientation, culture, ethnicity, socioeconomic status, educational attainment, religious affiliation
29. behavioral, marital, identification, and civic
30. race, ethnicity, gender, social class, or exceptionality
31. cultural awareness, cultural knowledge, cultural skills, cultural encounters, and cultural desires
32. vocabulary, grammatical structure, voice qualities, intonation, rhythm, speed, pronunciation, and silence
33. the use of silence, touch, eye movement, facial expressions, and body posture
34. secretiveness, shyness, guilt, lack of interest, or even a sign of mental illness
35. cultural preservation and maintenance, and cultural accommodation and negotiation
36. race, gender, sexual orientation, culture, ethnicity, socioeconomic status, educational attainment, religious affiliation
37. (1) If verbal communication cannot be established, developing a picture board for the client can be highly beneficial to meet the client's needs. Pictures of food, pills, doctor, bathroom, and so on can at least provide a basic form of communication. (2) To provide safe care, first establish a rapport with the client and the family who can help establish communication or an

understanding of what the client needs and how the goals will be met by both the nurse and the client. (3) Always address clients by their surnames (using Mr., Mrs., Ms., etc.) until they give you permission to address them by their given name. (4) Clients with language barriers will need to have interpreters to be able to explain medications and treatments. Family members may not be the best choice. Since they do not have medical backgrounds, they could misinterpret and create more problems.

38. d. *Rationale:* This is the only correct answer.
39. b. *Rationale:* All of these answers are similar but cultural diversity answers the question better than the others. Nurses should have a good understanding of ethnic differences, and it has only been lately that this was added to the nursing curriculum.
40. d. *Rationale:* We all protect our space, and even a client has a right to remain in his private space without being invaded. Nurses should explain and ask if it is OK to proceed with an examination or a procedure that is invasive.
41. b. *Rationale:* Our roots make us who we are. By understanding traditions that were passed down to us and are observed helps us to be more aware of the various cultures around us. Other cultures' traditions need to be honored to the best of our knowledge so not to offend or create more problems.
42. c. *Rationale:* Cultural mosaic is a term that describes how we can adopt beliefs from others yet maintain our own cultural beliefs and traditions.
43. d. *Rationale:* The U.S. Department of Health and Human Services strives to eliminate health disparities.
44. a. *Rationale:* Racial and Ethnic Approaches to Community Health (REACH) is the agency that strives to eliminate racial and ethnic disparities.
45. d. *Rationale:* Each area was founded by individuals with different cultures and backgrounds. Even though everything may look similar, they are different. We can go through a culture shock even in a distance of a couple of hundred miles. It can make a huge difference.
46. a. *Rationale:* A treatment strategy that is consistent with the client's beliefs may have a better chance of being successful.
47. b. *Rationale:* Communication is very important in nursing. In communicating with our clients, we can develop a plan that will fit into their cultures and customs. They will be more willing to follow such a plan.
48. b. *Rationale:* Nurses need to work with their clients and develop a plan of care that they will follow. Refusing to care for them and discharging them without addressing the health issues are not solutions. Documentation is necessary for all teaching, and cultural beliefs should be addressed and acknowledged. This also helps other nurses to find solutions to providing care that is not acceptable by their clients' culture.

Chapter 5

1. s   2. r   3. i   4. g   5. t   6. o
7. j   8. v   9. d   10. h   11. u   12. b
13. q   14. c   15. l   16. n   17. p   18. k
19. f   20. m   21. e   22. a

23. self-responsibility; an ultimate goal; a dynamic, growing process; daily decision making in the areas of nutrition, stress management, physical fitness, preventive health care, and emotional health; and the whole being of the individual
24. blood oxygen and carbon dioxide levels, blood pressure, body temperature, blood glucose, and fluid and electrolyte balance
25. self-regulating, compensatory, tend to be regulated by negative feedback systems, and may require several feedback mechanisms to correct only one physiologic imbalance
26. physiologic, safety and security, love and belonging, self-esteem, self-actualization
27. help clients monitor health, supply anticipatory guidance, impart knowledge about health, can reduce barriers to action, and support positive actions
28. genetic makeup, gender, age, and developmental level
29. age, sex, occupation, socioeconomic status, religion, ethnic origin, psychologic stability, personality, education, and modes of coping
30. information dissemination, health risk appraisal and wellness assessment, lifestyle and behavior change, and environmental control programs
31. mental, physical, emotional, spiritual, and environmental components
32. symptoms, sick role, medical care contact, dependent client role, and recovery or rehabilitation
33. behaviors, emotional state, attitudes, values, motives, abilities, habits, and appearances
34. appetite, rest and sleep pattern, energy level, sense of well-being, mood, usual activities, family relationships, and relationships with others
35. awareness, education, and growth
36. physical, spiritual, emotional, and intellectual
37. environment, culture, nutrition, safety, and many other elements
38. (1) Barb is experiencing nurse burnout. (2) When family or health problems arise, she would be eligible for the Family Leave Act. Since she has not had a vacation, she should be able to use her benefits to continue her paychecks while she is caring for her family. (3) Clients already have issues. If they perceive the nurse is not giving them their full attention, it will hinder their ability to concentrate on getting better and may even make them worse if they feel the nurse doesn't care. (4) Nurses and staff that have worked together for awhile usually try to support and help each other. They may even pass on their collective sick time to help her out financially.

39. c. *Rationale:* The body continues to change and requires energy to continually replace old dying cells with new ones.
40. b. *Rationale:* Sharing information leads to education, and through education comes better health.
41. d. *Rationale:* Guided imagery is a state of focus similar to hypnosis.
42. a. *Rationale:* Our bodies are over two-thirds water. Using hydrotherapy, whether hot or cold, provides relief for many ailments.
43. b. *Rationale:* Nurses need to teach clients how to stay well or how not to develop complications from existing problems. This helps keep them out of the hospital and also reduces the cost of health care.
44. d. *Rationale:* As with all employers, one of the costly expenses after orientation is absenteeism. When an employee is ill, someone else must take that person's place. This could be more costly and less efficient since the replacement will not have the knowledge about the position that the regular employee has.
45. c. *Rationale:* When we want to change something, we usually contemplate it and weigh the pros and cons.
46. a. *Rationale:* Time and energy is needed to put a plan into action.
47. c. *Rationale:* These stages are cyclical, but the termination stage is where the client has confidence the problem will no longer return.
48. b. *Rationale:* The nursing process, which consists of the other answers plus implementing and diagnosing, is the tool used by all nurses to care for clients.
49. b. *Rationale:* This is the most complete answer. The others can apply but NCLEX will always look for the answer that best fits the question.
50. c. *Rationale:* Health belief models were developed to improve health attitudes. Nurses need to encourage clients to live a healthier lifestyle through understanding and education.

Chapter 6

1. n 2. r 3. p 4. i 5. j 6. s
7. o 8. b 9. d 10. a 11. h 12. f
13. m 14. e 15. c 16. u 17. q 18. g
19. v 20. l 21. k 22. w 23. t
24. generating, implementing, and evaluating approaches for dealing with client care and professional concerns
25. use knowledge from other subjects and fields, deal with change in stressful environments, make important decisions, work as part of a team
26. critical thinking, problem solving, decision making
27. analysis, problem solving, decision making
28. assessing, diagnosing, planning, implementing, evaluating
29. technique to look beneath the surface, recognize and examine assumptions, search for inconsistencies, examine multiple points of view, and differentiate what one knows from what one believes
30. independence, fair-mindedness, insight, intellectual humility, intellectual courage, integrity, perseverance, confidence, and curiosity
31. identify the purpose, set the criteria, weight the criteria, seek alternatives, examine alternatives, project, implement, evaluate the outcome
32. age, culture, religion, socioeconomic levels, family structures
33. generate many ideas rapidly, are generally flexible and natural, create original solutions to problems, tend to be independent and self-confident, demonstrate individuality
34. reflection, context, dialogue, and time
35. look at advantages and disadvantages of each option, apply Maslow's hierarchy of needs, consider which tasks can be delegated to others, or use another priority-setting framework
36. cognitive ability, creativity, curiosity, interpersonal skills, cultural competence, psychomotor skills, and technological skills
37. (1) Critical-thinking skills have to be developed, but by working with other nurses and observing how they handle situations, graduate nurses learn how to solve issues that are similar. (2) The orienting nurse can give the graduate case studies to do on the clients and have the graduate work out "what if" problems using critical-thinking skills. (3) Teamwork is a concept that has worked and proven itself over time and will continue to provide the best client care. (4) Nursing schools need to constantly instruct and allow students to use critical-thinking skills in the classroom and in the clinical areas. Some are just starting to recognize that these skills are needed.
38. c. *Rationale:* The others listed are Greek philosophers but have nothing to do with a method of questioning.
39. b. *Rationale:* Clinical judgment is based on objective data, knowledge, and even past experiences. The other answers may contribute to the outcome. Narrative thinking helps make sense of a situation, analytic processes help generate alternative actions, and cognitive skills include decision making, problem solving, and critical thinking.
40. c. *Rationale:* The client is the nurse's responsibility and should be checked first. It's important that the equipment is operating OK. Once the client is checked, the nurse can trouble shoot to see what caused the alarm. It is always good to check electrical outlets at some time because the battery may run down but it is not the most crucial thing to check. Alarms are there for a reason and should not be ignored. Even a false alarm needs to be investigated.
41. d. *Rationale:* Use clinical thinking to anticipate outcomes and maintain safety for the client and the nurse. Responsibility is an obligation to act, but is not the key. Accountability is an obligation to answer

for the action. Professionalism is how others will perceive you.
42. b. *Rationale:* Nurses need to be safe practitioners by keeping the clients safe, reporting errors, and being accountable for their actions. Nurses are responsible for their actions. They should always appear and act professional. Safety is the key and helps to prevent errors. Nurses need to think one step ahead of the client's needs and be aware of things that can go wrong.
43. a. *Rationale:* Creative thinkers help generate new ideas to create original solutions independently. Decision makers help to form an idea. Advanced thinkers can help build on a solution but not create new ones. Critical thinkers are part of the process.
44. d. *Rationale:* This is the correct answer. The other answers help the process of critical thinking and are used to analyze situations. Inductive reasoning is part of the critical-thinking skills. Decision making is a critical-thinking process. Creative thinking helps generate new ideas.
45. c. *Rationale:* This is the best answer because problem solving clarifies the nature of the problem and suggests possible solutions. Deductive reasoning is reasoning from general to specific. In inductive reasoning, generalizations are formed from facts. Decision making is the application of a set of questions.
46. c. *Rationale*: A mind map helps the nurse to develop a plan that can be followed mentally step by step.
47. d. *Rationale:* Nurses are mandated to maintain skills and continue to learn through continuing education credits. Medical research is ongoing and changes are made faster than most can keep up with them, so it's important to read medical journals and attend seminars and skills fairs to stay on the cutting edge.
48. b. *Rationale:* Interpersonal skills are an important part of communication that will help nurses to have the knowledge to understand human behavior and social systems, and the ability to develop trusting relationships by listening and conveying compassion, interest, and information.

Chapter 7

1. f   2. r   3. w   4. h   5. t   6. s
7. i   8. y   9. c   10. l   11. n   12. o
13. x   14. q   15. m   16. g   17. a   18. d
19. k   20. j   21. v   22. u   23. p   24. e
25. b

26. assessing, diagnosing, planning, implementing, evaluating
27. initial assessment, problem-focused assessment, emergency assessment, and time-lapsed reassessment
28. health problems, related experience, health practices, values, and lifestyles
29. collecting data, organizing data, validating data, and documenting data
30. the nursing health history, physical assessment, primary care provider's history and physical examination, results of laboratory and diagnostic tests, and material contributed by other health personnel
31. sensations, feelings, values, beliefs, attitudes, and perception of personal health status and life situation
32. observing, interviewing, and examining
33. actual, risk, wellness, possible, and syndrome
34. young children, and clients who are confused, afraid, embarrassed, or distrustful, or do not speak the nurse's language
35. coping behaviors, health practices, previous illnesses, and allergies
36. to get or give information, identify problems of mutual concern, evaluate change, teach, provide support, or provide counseling or therapy
37. time, place, seating arrangement or distance, and language
38. inspection, auscultation, palpation, and percussion
39. start at the neck, thorax, abdomen, and extremities; and end at the toes
40. physiologic, self-concept, role function, and interdependence
41. (1) The nurse needs to involve social services to see why the client was allowed to be in such an uncared-for state and make arrangements for help when he is discharged. The nurse also needs to find a way to get him showered and to clean the wheelchair. The nurse can provide him with education about keeping himself clean and also changing positions to help prevent the reoccurrence of decubiti. (2) Collaboratively the nurse can work with the UAPs to get him cleaned up and send the chair to have the cleaning staff sanitize it. The nurse will also work with other staff members to collaborate on his care both preop and postop. (3) John will need help with ADLs. (4) Diagnoses would include impaired urinary elimination, impaired physical mobility, impaired tissue integrity, risk for infection, impaired skin integrity, self-care deficits—bathing/hygiene, and self-care deficits—toileting.
42. d. *Rationale:* The Joint Commission on Accreditation of Healthcare Organizations provides an accreditation for hospitals and mandates the way care is to be provided. The other answers have no bearing on this question.
43. c. *Rationale:* The first step of the nursing process is to assess, then plan, implement, and evaluate.
44. d. *Rationale:* Therapeutic communication is purposeful and client focused, which is important in working with clients. Social communication is a safe way to communicate but will not benefit the client, and structured communication is used for interviewing.
45. b. *Rationale:* Psychomotor skills involve physical action. All the other answers have only the first few letters in common.
46. d. *Rationale:* The last phase is evaluation but this is never the final phase unless the nursing diagnosis is

resolved. The other phases are all prior to an evaluation.
47. a. *Rationale:* Evaluating and assessing overlap and are continuous once a nurse evaluates a client's progress. They need to be reassessed and the process continues with every client contact. The other phases are important. Without the implementing phase in which the plan is put into action, there would be nothing to evaluate.
48. c. *Rationale:* The planning step helps to get to the desired outcomes while the other steps function to build on the process.
49. d. *Rationale:* The evaluation statement shows that the outcome was met and the client's responses support it. The other answers are part of the nursing process.
50. a. *Rationale:* This is part of professional accountability. Nurses are responsible and accountable for their actions. The other answers are also important parts of the medical profession but have nothing to do with this question.
51. b. *Rationale:* The nursing process with its five phases is a fluid process that helps nurses to approach client care from an organized manner. The other answers are phases in that process.
52. a. *Rationale:* Subjective data could be things the client feels that are not measurable, such as a headache or nausea. Objective data can be measured, such as vomit or blood or a wound.
53. c. *Rationale:* Discharge is planned when the client is admitted and is evaluated every day so the final plan is completed when the client is ready to go home or be transferred to another facility.
54. b. *Rationale:* This plan reflects the client's specific needs that may not apply to all clients with those diagnoses, making it individualized.
55. b. *Rationale:* If clients have no identifiable problems, the nurse needs to concentrate on health promotion to maintain and improve their health.

Chapter 8

1. b   2. d   3. t   4. s   5. p   6. h
7. j   8. r   9. m   10. k   11. o   12. n
13. l   14. c   15. q   16. i   17. a   18. f
19. e   20. g

21. communication, planning client care, auditing health agencies, research, education, reimbursement, legal documentation, health care analysis
22. timely, complete, accurate, confidential, and specific to the client
23. comprehensive view of the client, the illness, effective treatment strategies, and factors that affect the outcome of the illness
24. the source-oriented record; the problem-oriented medical record; the problems, interventions, evaluation (PIE) model; focus charting; charting by exception (CBE); computerized documentation; and case management
25. the database, the problem list, the plan of care, and the progress notes
26. subjective data, objective data, assessment, and planning
27. specific problems, mental status, ADLs, hydration and nutrition status, safety measures, medications, treatments, preventive measures, and behavioral modifications assessment as needed
28. management information systems and hospital information systems
29. professional education for nursing students and clients; assessing, documenting, and testing clients' health conditions; managing medical records; communicating among health care providers and with clients; and conducting nursing research
30. recording of client assessments, medication administration, progress notes, care plan updating, client acuity, and accrued charges
31. constant availability of client health information across the life span, ability to monitor quality, access to warehoused (stored) data, and ability for clients to share in knowledge and activities influencing their own health
32. client's name and medical diagnosis, changes in nursing assessment, vital signs related to baseline vital signs, significant laboratory data, and related nursing interventions
33. problems, interventions, and evaluation
34. evidence of client assessments, nursing diagnoses and/or client needs, nursing interventions, client outcomes, and evidence of a current nursing care plan
35. (a) A comprehensive assessment (the Minimum Data Set [MDS] for Resident Assessment and Care Screening) must be performed within four days of a client's admission to a long-term care facility, (b) a formulated plan of care must be completed within seven days of admission, and (c) the assessment and care screening process must be reviewed every three months.
36. chemotherapy, tube feedings, and ventilators
37. (1) Since clients' charts are legal documents, the nurse must make the corrections to them. If the charts are no longer on the unit, she can go to the medical records department and make the corrections before they are microfilmed and send the corrected chart to the long-term care facility. (2) Corrections need to be done by drawing a single line through the mistake, writing "mistaken entry" over it, and then initialing it. (3) There is no excuse for not completing charts, and the nurse could be in jeopardy of losing her job if she does not do the documentation. (4) If the chart were to go to court and those entries were believed to be true, it could create issues for the client. At the long-term care facility, it could be confusing when they review the chart.
38. a. *Rationale:* DRGs established a coding system to equate payments for services paid for by the insurance

and to reduce the cost of health care for Medicare and third-party payers.
39. b. *Rationale:* Focus charting is the only one that is holistic.
40. d. *Rationale:* Of the many charting systems, only case management is multidisciplinary and uses the critical pathways. The others are basic charting systems used in hospitals.
41. c. *Rationale:* Charting by exception looks at the problems and can track changes in the client's condition.
42. b. *Rationale:* Case management uses the critical pathways. The other answers are systems used for charting client information.
43. d. *Rationale*: Clients' charts are legal documents and can be subpoenaed to go to court. The best way is to draw a line through the mistake so it can still be read and then write "mistaken entry" and initial it. The other answers are illegal and could create legal problems.
44. c. *Rationale:* The use of fax machines actually started the HIPAA movement when faxes were sent to the wrong numbers and sensitive medical information was leaked. The cover sheets were added so that if it is sent to the wrong machine it should be destroyed and not read. The other answers are part of the fax but not the most important.
45. d. *Rationale:* The framework and steps in the nursing process and doing complete charting will keep nurses out of trouble.
46. c. *Rationale:* PDAs are often used in facilities to chart immediately and can send results back to a mainframe. The other answers are other electronic devices.
47. d. *Rationale:* ANA (American Nurses Association) set up the code of ethics. HIPAA is the act that protects clients' privacy and rights to provide information or not. OBRA has more influence over long-term care facilities. JCAHO is the accrediting body for hospitals.
48. c. *Rationale:* These are all part of PIE, but the disadvantage is reviewing all the notes to determine which problems are current and which interventions were effective.
49. a. *Rationale:* Case management uses graphics and flow sheets and promotes collaboration and teamwork. It also helps to decrease length of stay, and makes efficient use of time.

Chapter 9

1. c   2. t   3. w   4. b   5. u   6. a
7. d   8. l   9. e   10. f   11. s   12. g
13. k   14. i   15. j   16. h   17. m   18. p
19. v   20. n   21. x   22. q   23. o   24. r
25. height, weight, bone size, and dentition
26. psychosocial, moral, spiritual, and cognitive advances
27. genetics, temperament, family, nutrition, environmental, health, cultural
28. concepts of the unconscious mind, defense mechanisms, and the id, ego, and superego
29. trust versus mistrust, autonomy versus shame and doubt, initiative versus guilt, industry versus inferiority, identity versus role confusion, intimacy versus isolation, generativity versus stagnation, integrity versus despair
30. oral, anal, phallic, genital
31. the sensorimotor phase, the preconceptual phase, the intuitive thought phase, the concrete operations phase, and the formal operations phase
32. identification, introjection, imagination, and repression
33. motor vehicle crashes, other unintentional injuries (falls, drowning, poisoning), suicides, and homicide
34. Freud, Havighurst, Piaget, Vygotsky, Gould, Skinner, Erikson
35. being sensitive to the infant's needs and meeting these needs promptly and skillfully, responding consistently to an infant's needs, and providing a predictable environment in which routines are established
36. psychosocial, cognitive, moral, spiritual, and behavioral aspects
37. temperament, feelings, character traits, independence, self-esteem, self-concept, behavior, ability to interact with others, and ability to adapt to life changes
38. activity level, sensitivity, intensity, adaptability, distractibility, approach/withdrawal, mood, persistence, regularity
39. (1) Initiative versus guilt is the developmental stage for 3- to 5-year-olds. (2) She has regressed to autonomy versus shame and doubt, causing her to go back to the bed-wetting stage. (3) By providing love and attention and working with her as she gets well, her mother will help her to move to the stage she was in and to prepare to move to the next stage. (4) Depending on the age of the person and how entrenched he or she is into the stage, serious traumas can definitely move a person back even several stages, especially with head trauma.
40. c. *Rationale:* The ego is the realistic part of the person's mind balancing the gratification demands of the id.
41. b. *Rationale:* Erikson worked on Freud's original theory and expanded it. The other theorists have also made contributions but nurses need to understand these stages to gauge where a client is in terms of development.
42. d. *Rationale:* Erikson's stages were developed to follow a sequence. Each level must be accomplished or the person can be stuck in that level forever.
43. b. *Rationale:* Havighurst explained what developmental stages are and also developed six stages.
44. c. *Rationale:* Peck felt the body aged but the mind improved.
45. d. *Rationale:* Piaget developed the theory of cognitive development. The other theorists developed similar theories or built on Piaget's theory.

46. a. *Rationale:* Infants who do not gain weight and grow are diagnosed as failure to thrive.
47. a. *Rationale:* Defense mechanisms are used as a socially acceptable manner for the ego to fulfill the id. The other answers are personality traits.
48. c. *Rationale:* The genital stage promotes energy that is directed toward sexual maturity and developing skills to cope with the environment. The other answers are earlier stages.
49. a. *Rationale:* Robert Havighurst used the developmental theory and felt that learning is a concept that continues throughout the lifespan. The other theorists have also developed developmental theories.
50. d. *Rationale:* Infants require all of their needs to be met.
51. a. *Rationale:* Libido changes its location of emphasis within the body from one stage to another, making that area more important at a given time.
52. c. *Rationale:* When the client has not met a developmental stage and is behind, the nurse can give the client opportunities to be successful in the stage he or she is currently in.
53. b. *Rationale:* Although these all seem similar, reasoning is what Kohlberg was theorizing and that few reach the highest level.

Chapter 10

1. d 2. g 3. i 4. l 5. c 6. m
7. a 8. k 9. f 10. b 11. e 12. h
13. j
14. provider of care, teacher, manager, advocate, and research consumer
15. a great deal of patience, expertise, understanding, interdisciplinary communication, and compassion skills
16. acute care hospital, subacute or transitional care, and long-term care facilities
17. genetics, oxidative stress, cellular changes
18. lean body mass is reduced, fat tissue increases, and bone mass decreases
19. smoking cessation, maintaining ideal body weight, exercising daily, avoiding foods high in sodium and fat and eating fruits and vegetables, and discussing the use of low-dose aspirin therapy with the primary provider
20. sugar, caffeine, alcohol, chocolate, artificial sweeteners, and spicy and acidic foods
21. sense of continuity, family heritage, rituals, and folklore
22. substance abuse, incarceration, teen pregnancy, emotional problems, and parental death
23. perception, cognitive agility, memory, and learning
24. cultural background, life experiences, gender, religion, and socioeconomic status
25. advancements in disease control, living conditions, and health technology
26. gender, marital status, education, income, and living arrangements
27. healthy diet, physical activity, stress management
28. (1) Older clients today can stay in their own homes with the help of visiting nursing groups, life alert monitors, modifications to the home to make them more accessible, and even services that will take them to appointments or shopping. (2) She should be checked by a physician to address the issues, but weight loss is common with the elderly. Medications often make foods taste different or they just lose their appetites. (3) We do label them and tend to think all elderly are the same, but with the technology and medical advances we have today some elderly age more gracefully than others. If they stay active, they do not have the stereotypical problems we saw with the elderly years ago. (4) Her best option would depend on her lifestyle. Many of the retirement homes offer apartments where you live alone but can meet in common areas for meals and socialization. Her family could invite her for visits and she could look into a retirement center.
29. c. *Rationale:* Income is inversely compared to the level of education.
30. b. *Rationale:* Hearing loss is known as presbycusis. Presbyopia is the loss of visual acuity, and Presbyterian is a form of religion.
31. c. *Rationale:* Kohlberg felt that a person defines good and bad in relation to self, whereas older people at stage 2 may act to meet another's needs as well as their own.
32. a. *Rationale:* Gilligan challenged Kohlberg's theory and felt women and men have different moral standards.
33. b. *Rationale:* Nurses are responsible to report any abuse whether it is a child or the elderly.
34. b. *Rationale:* Although many forms of dementia are being diagnosed, Alzheimer's is the most common. NPH has also shown an increased diagnosis but is often missed by the physician as a viable diagnosis.
35. d. *Rationale:* Spirituality is often at a higher level in the elderly because they were brought up in a different era. The other answers are possible but this is the best answer.
36. c. *Rationale:* The older population are the ones who suffer from health issues that crop up with age, regardless of lifestyle. These can be strokes or heart attacks.
37. d. *Rationale:* This is the best answer although some may think other answers are equally as good.
38. a. *Rationale:* Although most of these statements could apply, the cause and effect would be falls (which can result in fractures) or pathologic fractures (which could actually occur first and then lead to a fall if the person has osteoporosis).
39. a. *Rationale:* The nurse should be aware of whether medications that are administered are excreted via the kidney or liver and if the client show signs of toxicity.

40. d. *Rationale:* Timing, because it takes longer to become sexually aroused, longer to complete intercourse, and longer before sexual arousal can occur again.
41. c. *Rationale:* If older persons have followed and completed Erikson's tasks, they will feel good about their lives and what they have accomplished.

Chapter 11

1. i   2. g   3. f   4. e   5. a   6. d
7. b   8. c   9. h

10. the individual, the family, and the community
11. male or female, youth or adult, legally or not legally related, genetically or not genetically related
12. physical activity, weight management, abstinence from substance abuse, responsible sexual behaviors, and maintaining immunization status
13. married couples with children, married couples without children, other family households (single-parent families), men living alone, women living alone, and other nonfamily households
14. death of a spouse, separation, divorce, birth of a child to an unmarried woman, or adoption of a child by a single man or woman
15. child care concerns, financial concerns, role overload and fatigue in managing daily tasks, and social isolation
16. neurologic, musculoskeletal, respiratory, circulatory, gastrointestinal, and urinary subsystems
17. developing a sense of family purpose and affiliation, adding and socializing new members, and providing and distributing care and services to members
18. clarify family interaction patterns, identify family strengths and weaknesses, and describe the health status of the family and its individual members
19. maturity level of individual family members, heredity or genetic factors, sex or race, sociologic factors, and lifestyle practices
20. cancers, cardiovascular disease, adult-onset diabetes, and tooth decay
21. support, understanding, and encouragement
22. family's structure, methods of interaction, health care practices, and coping mechanisms
23. live in houses, apartments, urban areas, rural towns; some are homeless
24. (1) The nurse should be on the lookout for abuse. (2) The nurse should ask how the injury occurred and see if the child gives the same answer and if the injury could have occurred in the way it is being explained. (3) The nurse should look at the time line when they arrived in America since the injuries could have happened while they were living in Iraq as a product of the war. Another consideration is whether that culture permits parents to physically punish their children. (4) It probably is safer to have social services involved just to err on the side of safety. It would provide an opportunity for the family to have an understanding on the rights of children and the laws in their new country.
25. b. *Rationale:* Acculturation is needed to allow families to grasp and understand the norms of the new culture.
26. c. *Rationale:* Many cultures have all family members living in the same house. With the tight economy, it is cheaper and actually better for the family to all live together. The young can learn from the old, and grandparents can care for the children while the parents work.
27. a. *Rationale:* Cohabitating allows for non-family members to live together. Many households are blended so that expenses can be shared to provide a quality of life for the group.
28. d. *Rationale:* Ludwig von Bertalanffy is the only correct answer. The others worked on developmental theories.
29. a. *Rationale:* These are all processes that the body works through, but feedback is the basic input-output system.
30. c. *Rationale:* Family-centered care is important for the client and for the family since each builds on the other. Family members can contribute information and provide care before and after discharge.
31. b. *Rationale:* Groups of like cultures can isolate themselves by not mingling with others. They also may not develop language skills normal for the region and can cluster into one region and develop a mini city within a city.
32. d. *Rationale:* Although we rarely see this type of traditional family, it used to be the norm. Today we actually see more women working and men staying home.
33. c. *Rationale:* Some states have passed legislation that identifies same-sex couples as having the same rights as married people.
34. b. *Rationale:* Although some of these answers are also part of Johnson's work, this is the best answer.
35. a. *Rationale:* It focuses on intrafamily relationships with the structure and function.

Chapter 12

1. d   2. e   3. f   4. b   5. g   6. a
7. c

8. knowing, alternating rhythms, patience, honesty, trust, humility, hope, courage
9. caring as a moral imperative, affect, human trait, interpersonal relationship, therapeutic intervention
10. compassion, competence, confidence, conscience, commitment, and comportment
11. empathy, compassion, holism, and sensitivity
12. diversity of human responses, the nurse's workload, and the preferences of the nurse and client
13. by being true to self, being real, and being who they truly are

14. protection, enhancement, and preservation of human dignity
15. to health-illness conditions; a knowledge of health-illness, environmental-personal interactions; a knowledge of the nurse caring process; self-knowledge, knowledge of one's power and transaction limitations
16. empirical knowledge, personal knowing, ethical knowing, aesthetic knowing
17. conservation of life, alleviation of suffering, and promotion of health
18. by using an appropriate pain scale, the client's positioning, hygiene, amount of rest, and other physiologic variables
19. coaching, informing, explaining, supporting, assisting, guiding, focusing, and validating
20. (1) People working in all professions can get burned out. If you become burned out as a nurse, you need to take a vacation and reevaluate what you want to do. (2) Nursing is a profession that helps you fulfill yourself as you provide care for others. It is such a great feeling to see a client improve enough to be discharged. (3) It is difficult for schools to select students who will make good nurses. Students who fulfill the criteria are given a chance to go through the program. (4) Having goals is important in any profession, but especially in nursing where furthering education and using skills mastered can lead to many advantages in promoting new careers. A ten year goal is important to know where you are headed.
21. a. *Rationale:* She felt caring is one of the most critical factors in helping people regain health. The others are nursing theorists who focused on caring.
22. d. *Rationale:* She based her studies on nursing and anthropology and noted that caring as nurturing behavior has been present throughout history. The others are nursing theorists who focused on caring.
23. b. *Rationale:* Mayeroff felt by helping the other grow, the caregiver moves toward self-actualization.
24. d. *Rationale:* His theory of bureaucratic caring focuses on caring in organizations.
25. d. *Rationale:* In switching places the nurse and client can identify with each other. The nurse and client gain self-knowledge and keep alive their common humanity.
26. a. *Rationale:* Nurses are there for the clients. They answer bells and are ever vigilant in meeting the needs and being present.
27. d. *Rationale:* Nurses need to lead the way to better health and prevention through healthy lifestyles. Holistic nurses strive to achieve that harmony in their own lives and to assist others who are striving to do the same.
28. c. *Rationale:* Unfortunately, being a caring person has to be developed and no amount of education can make someone care. Student nurses need to reflect on a practice that must be personal and meaningful.
29. b. *Rationale:* A mentor is a guide who has attained a goal such as nursing and now teaches it and works to pass knowledge on to other nursing students. Students who have mentors do much better in the clinical areas through the hands-on guidance of another.

Chapter 13

1. f 2. i 3. l 4. m 5. a 6. j
7. e 8. n 9. b 10. h 11. d 12. o
13. k 14. g 15. c
16. influence others and obtain information
17. collect assessment data, initiate interventions, evaluate outcomes of interventions, initiate change that promotes health, and prevent legal problems associated with nursing practice
18. a sender, a message, a receiver, and a response
19. verbal and nonverbal
20. includes gestures, body movements, use of touch, and physical appearance
21. surprise, fear, anger, disgust, happiness, and sadness
22. the development of trust and acceptance between the nurse and the client, and an underlying belief that the nurse cares about and wants to help the client
23. age, sex, appearance, diagnosis, education, values, ethnic and cultural background, personality, expectations, and the setting
24. The client should develop trust in the nurse; view the nurse as a competent professional capable of helping; view the nurse as honest, open, and concerned about the client's welfare; believe the nurse will try to understand and respect the client's cultural values and beliefs; believe the nurse will respect client confidentiality; feel comfortable talking with the nurse about feelings and other sensitive issues; understand the purpose of the relationship and the roles; and feel that the nurse and client are active participants in developing a mutually agreeable plan of care.
25. exploring and understanding thoughts and feelings, and facilitating and taking action
26. to gather assessment data, to teach and persuade, and to express caring and comfort
27. pace, intonation, simplicity, clarity, brevity, timing, relevance, adaptability, credibility, and humor
28. (1) The NANDA diagnosis for the communication could be *Fear* or *Anxiety*. (2) The medical diagnosis could be early onset of Alzheimer's or normal pressure hydrocephalus. (3) The wife first needs a definitive diagnosis and how to care for him. (4) Communicating with a client who has a short attention span and is defiant will take some work. The nurse should try to find an area of trust and understanding and then build on the relationship to hopefully create a bond. Methods might include manipulating the environment, providing support, employing measures to enhance communication, and educating the client and support person.

29. c. *Rationale:* Encoding is the correct answer.
30. b. *Rationale:* E-mail is mail sent electronically. Faxes are also electronic but e-mail is the most used form.
31. d. *Rationale:* Nurses communicate with their clients and do a great deal of explaining and teaching. Without attentive listening by both the sender and the receiver the message will not get across.
32. b. *Rationale:* An aggressive form of action or communication can often include screaming, sarcasm, rudeness, belittling jokes, and even direct personal insults.
33. b. *Rationale:* Nurses should find a way to communicate with the client since they will be providing the care. If the client can blink for yes and no answers, the nurse will have a good idea if the client understands.
34. a. *Rationale:* Nurses are narrative and try to tell the physician the facts, and the physician basically looks at the issues.
35. c. *Rationale:* Although technically all the answers could work, the best is to know your style by listening to yourself.
36. b. *Rationale:* Open-ended questions will allow more information to be exchanged between the sender and the receiver.
37. d. *Rationale:* Although all of these components are important, speaking slowly and enunciating are the most important.
38. c. *Rationale:* The best way to know what is happening with the client would be to ask the client directly.
39. a. *Rationale:* With a total message, nurses should be aware of what the client says and the body language that the client displays.
40. a. *Rationale:* To trust another person involves risk, but in order to have an open relationship you must take the risk.
41. b. *Rationale:* Nurses need to be able to put themselves in their clients' shoes to have a better understanding of how they feel about their situation. The other answers are also important but empathy works the best.

Chapter 14

1. g 2. j 3. f 4. o 5. k 6. q
7. a 8. c 9. l 10. e 11. m 12. r
13. p 14. h 15. d 16. n 17. i 18. s
19. b
20. the literacy level, educational background, language skills, and culture of every client
21. promoting, protecting, and maintaining health
22. The process communicates information, emotions, perceptions, and attitudes to the other.
23. As people mature, they move from dependence to independence. An adult's previous experiences can be used as a resource for learning. An adult's readiness to learn is often related to a developmental task or social role. An adult is more oriented to learning when the material is useful immediately, not sometime in the future.
24. behaviorism, cognitivism, and humanism
25. sensorimotor phase, the preconceptual phase, the intuitive phase, the concrete operations phase, and the formal operations phase
26. change in cognitive structure, change in motivation, change in one's sense of belonging to the group, and gain in voluntary muscle control
27. unfreezing, moving, and refreezing
28. cognitive, affective, and psychomotor
29. support of desired behavior through praise, positively worded corrections, and suggestions of alternative methods
30. cultural, physiologic events, emotions, psychomotor abilities
31. knowing, comprehending, and applying to analysis, synthesis, and evaluation
32. (1) The nurse can help by using support groups or by having a person who has gone through it to speak with him. (2) If the client will not look at or touch his colostomy, using a model may be helpful since it is not soiled and not a part of him. (3) Social services could help to provide care in the home so he can be discharged and they can continue to teach and encourage him to care for himself. (4) The wife should be taught how to care for the colostomy, but only as a backup. The client needs to meet his own needs as he did before the colostomy.
33. d. *Rationale:* JCAHO accredits hospitals and sets up standards for client care. The others are agencies who also contribute to the best care of clients.
34. c. *Rationale:* Thorndike believed that learners' behaviors contributed to their ability to learn.
35. a. *Rationale:* Bandura believed in observation rather than trial and error. The others are also behavior theorists.
36. b. *Rationale:* Learning styles are effective to provide information to clients that they will use to improve their health. The other answers are all part of understanding a client by knowing how he lives and who provides him with support.
37. c. *Rationale:* The best answer is that clients will not seek help for their health issues. The other answers should all be the opposite. Literacy issues create more problems and cost taxpayers more money because clients do not seek help when they first detect a problem.
38. b. *Rationale:* Usually they are embarrassed that they cannot read, so they do not let anyone know that they have a problem.
39. a. *Rationale:* Placing a nursing diagnosis on the client's care plan will alert other nurses to the problem and they will be able to work around the issue and provide the tools that the client can use to learn.

40. b. *Rationale:* Clients should take responsibility for their own care, so checking the orders once they get home will help them to be compliant and understand.
41. c. *Rationale:* In health care literature, adherence is commitment or attachment to a regimen. Nurses determine if the client can and will be compliant and can adhere to the teaching to maintain health.
42. c. *Rationale:* Bloom's taxonomy is the only answer that is correct for this question.
43. c. *Rationale:* Students need to be motivated to learn. In learning they promote change, and as they change they become more motivated.
44. a. *Rationale:* The plan must be revised when the client's needs change or the teaching strategies prove ineffective.

Chapter 15

1. u 2. h 3. a 4. w 5. r 6. l
7. d 8. p 9. n 10. f 11. b 12. q
13. j 14. t 15. z 16. y 17. s 18. k
19. o 20. g 21. m 22. i 23. v 24. x
25. e 26. c

27. leadership, management, delegation, and change
28. informed, articulate, confident, self-aware, outstanding interpersonal skills, excellent listeners and communicators
29. improving the health status of individuals or families, increasing the effectiveness and level of satisfaction among professional colleagues, and improving the attitudes of citizens and legislators toward the nursing profession and their expectations of it
30. good judgment, decisiveness, knowledge, adaptability, integrity, tact, self-confidence, and cooperativeness
31. autocratic, democratic, laissez-faire, and bureaucratic
32. efficiently accomplishing the goals of the organization; efficiently using the organization's resources; ensuring effective client care; and ensuring compliance with institutional, professional, regulatory, and governmental standards
33. flexes task and relationship behaviors, considers the staff members' abilities, knows the nature of the task to be done, and is sensitive to the context or environment in which the task takes place
34. requires an understanding of factors such as needs, goals, and rewards that motivate people; knowledge of leadership skills and of the group's activities; possession of the interpersonal skills to influence others; vision; influence; and acting as a role model
35. thought, care, insight, commitment, and energy
36. planning, organizing, directing, coordinating, communicating, managing resources, enhancing employee performance, building and managing teams
37. anticipating and seeking sources of risk; analyzing, classifying, and prioritizing risks; developing a plan to avoid and manage risk; gathering data that indicate success at avoiding or minimizing risk; and evaluating and modifying risk reduction programs
38. think critically, communicate well, manage resources effectively and efficiently, enhance employee performance, build and manage teams, manage conflict, manage time, and initiate and manage change
39. (1) A preceptor works with new graduates. (2) The manager seems to be a laissez-faire manager. (3) The preceptor offers many years of experience and will provide the graduate with guidance. (4) Many skills are learned during clinical rotations, but some things are not available when students are on the units. Lists of skills should include a safe way to dispense medications and do basic dressing changes and procedures that are carried out on the unit.
40. c. *Rationale:* A democratic leader allows for self-motivation and creativity as well as a great deal of cooperation and coordination among group members.
41. c. *Rationale:* Each state nurse practice act specifies which actions constitute the legal practice of nursing, which actions are the purview only of nurses, and which may be delegated to others. The other agencies contribute to the nursing profession.
42. a. *Rationale:* Change agents use their problem-solving skills to gain new knowledge or adapt what is currently known. The other answers are similar but not the best answers.
43. b. *Rationale:* This is the only correct answer.
44. d. *Rationale:* Change is progress. Things will change every day, hopefully for the better. The best answer is d although all the other answers could also work.
45. d. *Rationale:* Usually unlicensed personnel cannot delegate to others but there may be instances that they can delegate to other like staff if they have more experience and are sure the other person is capable to carry out the task.
46. c. *Rationale:* Influence is exercised through persuasion and excellent communication skills; it is based on a trusting relationship with the followers.
47. a. *Rationale:* Most people want things to stay as they are because it can be frustrating to learn how to do something differently. For the masses, change is not accepted.
48. d. *Rationale:* Leaders work and manage people while managers are responsible for staying on budget and keeping all needed items available.

Chapter 16

1. j 2. t 3. u 4. hh 5. h 6. k
7. v 8. c 9. ii 10. w 11. f 12. y
13. p 14. r 15. x 16. e 17. d 18. z
19. n 20. g 21. l 22. i 23. o 24. q
25. a 26. m 27. dd 28. cc 29. s 30. gg
31. ff 32. aa 33. b 34. ee 35. bb 36. jj

37. temperature, pulse, respirations, blood pressure, pain

38. basal metabolic rate, muscle activity, thyroxine output, epinephrine, norepinephrine, and sympathetic stimulation/stress response
39. radiation, conduction, convection, and vaporization
40. sensors in the shell and in the core, an integrator in the hypothalamus, and an effector system that adjusts the production and loss of heat
41. shivering increases heat production, sweating is inhibited to decrease heat loss, and vasoconstriction decreases heat loss
42. age, diurnal variations, exercise, hormones, stress, and environment
43. inadequate diet, loss of subcutaneous fat, lack of activity, and reduced thermoregulatory efficiency
44. intermittent, remittent, relapsing, and constant
45. clients who are undergoing rectal surgery, have diarrhea or diseases of the rectum, are immunosuppressed, have a clotting disorder, or have significant hemorrhoids
46. age, gender, exercise, fever, medication, hypovolemia, stress, position change, pathology
47. temporal, carotid, radial, femoral, pedal, popliteal, brachial, posterior tibia, apical
48. (1) The client is suffering from orthostatic hypotension. (2) All medical personnel should understand that they need to use the appropriate size equipment to receive an accurate reading. (3) By using a smaller cuff, it would give a higher reading. (4) They should have checked her BP with a cuff that fits and do BPs both sitting and standing to see if it drops when she stands up.
49. d. *Rationale:* This part of the brain controls the temperature with checks and balances.
50. d. *Rationale:* The apical pulse is a central pulse located at the apex of the heart. This is the most noted since the heart controls the peripheral pulses and helps to evaluate the heart for disease.
51. c. *Rationale*: A heart rate 100 or more is called tachycardia. Bradycardia is a slow heart rate, and the other terms are related to the respiratory system.
52. d. *Rationale:* The Korotkoff's sounds may or may not be audible, but this is the best answer. Even though d is similar, it does not give as much information.
53. a. *Rationale:* Although all answers are correct, the best one explains the damage to the brain and this can cause death.
54. d. *Rationale:* The only information given is vital signs, and they should be correlated with age, gender, and often a baseline, but given this information the high temperature with all other signs lower would be indicative of septic shock.
55. c. *Rationale:* Orthostatic hypotension is the term used for a BP that drops with position changes caused by peripheral vasodilatation.
56. b. *Rationale:* By placing a small sensor to an index finger, it will give a reading for oxygen saturation and should be greater than 90. The other items are not for measuring oxygen.
57. d. *Rationale:* The oral route is the most common and especially with electronic equipment is the safest if there are no issues with the mouth. The tympanic is equivalent to an oral temperature, but one of the problems is that if the thermometer is not properly inserted the reading will not be accurate. The rectal is invasive and can create other problems such as vagal stimulation. The axillary would be at least one degree off and also invasive, especially for females.
58. c. *Rationale:* Wet clothes should be removed and replaced with dry ones so the body temperature does not drop below a safe range. Wet clothes could cause chafing but that is not a medical problem. It is doubtful that wet clothes would cause hyperthermia or hypotension.
59. c. *Rationale:* Arms are often off limits due to IVs, lymphadema, cellulitis, fractures, and so on. When this happens the next choice would be to use the thigh and the popliteal artery.
60. a. *Rationale:* The direct method is an invasive procedure that gives an accurate blood pressure.

Chapter 17

1. s 2. i 3. j 4. x 5. c 6. a
7. m 8. q 9. g 10. e 11. o 12. r
13. w 14. y 15. z 16. t 17. h 18. l
19. k 20. n 21. v 22. f 23. p 24. u
25. d 26. b

27. a complete assessment (e.g., when a client is admitted to a health care agency); examination of a body system (e.g., the cardiovascular system); or examination of a body area such as lung sounds
28. obtain baseline data, verify data obtained in the nursing history, obtain data that will contribute to the nursing diagnosis and plan of care, evaluate client outcomes and response to treatment, make clinical judgments about health status, and identify areas for health promotion and illness prevention
29. inspection, palpation, percussion, and auscultation
30. gowning and/or draping the client appropriately, positioning the client comfortably, and ensuring that their own hands are warm before beginning
31. location, distribution, configuration, color, shape, size, firmness, texture, and characteristics of individual lesions
32. the client's chief complaints; the client's physical condition, because many parts of the examination require movement and coordination of the extremities; and the client's willingness to participate and cooperate
33. mental status, including level of consciousness; the cranial nerves; reflexes; motor function; and sensory function
34. eye response, motor response, and verbal response
35. the biceps reflex, the triceps reflex, the brachioradialis reflex, the patellar reflex, the Achilles reflex, and the plantar reflex

36. helps to control posture, acts with the cerebral cortex to make body movements smooth and coordinated, and controls skeletal muscles to maintain equilibrium
37. client complaints, the nurse's own observation of problems, the client's presenting problem, nursing interventions provided, and medical therapies
38. flatness, dullness, resonance, hyperresonance, and tympany
39. brittleness, discoloration, thickening, distortion of nail shape, crumbling of the nail, and loosening of the nail
40. right upper quadrant, left upper quadrant, right lower quadrant, and left lower quadrant
41. (1) The symptoms could point to diabetes and the nurse could do a urine check for glucose and also do a chemstrip. (2) The physician should know all the symptoms and the chief complaints. (3) The nurse should get a detailed family history, especially if anyone in the family has diabetes. (4) He will need to change his diet and be instructed to check his glucose.
42. b. *Rationale:* Auscultation is listening. The other terms are used for the touch and visualizing during an exam.
43. d. *Rationale:* The test is also known as a Pap smear or Pap test, but Papanicolaou test is the proper term.
44. c. *Rationale:* Most women doing breast exams often do not go far enough. They need to check the axilla area. All other areas should also be checked monthly, but the tail of Spence is at the axilla.
45. b. *Rationale:* The best light to use is natural. The other forms are common ways that light an office. Black light is used to look for body fluids by CSI teams.
46. d. *Rationale:* The only definitive place is the eyes. The other areas, although they may be lighter, will not show jaundice until later if at all.
47. c. *Rationale:* Checking the skin turgor is the best way. Checking urine may be a late sign, and assessing mucous membranes is not definitive since medications can cause dry mouth.
48. d. *Rationale:* A zinc deficiency creates white spots on the nails. Iron deficiency causes spoon-like ridges.
49. b. *Rationale:* This is normal for the average person. The other answers are not correct.
50. b. *Rationale:* The thyroid, unless diseased, is not visible. This is the only answer that is correct.
51. a. *Rationale:* This is the only correct answer.
52. a. *Rationale:* Earpieces not only need to be comfortable, but they also need to be inserted in a way that promotes the best sound. Nurses should also check to make sure the earpiece is on tight so as not to puncture an eardrum.
53. c. *Rationale:* Using senses, especially olfactory senses, can help diagnose problems and may help to improve the health of the client. An example could be the smell of *Pseudomonas,* which is often found in a tracheostomy and has a very distinctive odor.
54. c. *Rationale:* An in-grown nail is known as paronychia.
55. d. *Rationale:* Plaque consists of bacteria, molecules of saliva, and remnants of epithelial cells and leukocyte. If left it forms tartar and causes teeth to decay.
56. c. *Rationale:* Rickets is a lack of vitamin D. A protruding sternum characterizes pigeon chest.
57. a. *Rationale:* When two bones rub together, usually at a joint such as knee, hip, and shoulder, it is called crepitation. This is a result of arthritis.

Chapter 18

1. e   2. k   3. n   4. q   5. a   6. r
7. l   8. o   9. s   10. d   11. m   12. t
13. w   14. b   15. y   16. h   17. j   18. g
19. v   20. x   21. z   22. c   23. f   24. u
25. p   26. i

27. insomnia, weight gain, constipation, hypertension, deconditioning, chronic stress, and depression
28. work, recreation, domestic activities, and personal care activities
29. promote healing, prevent complications, reduce suffering, and prevent the development of incurable pain states
30. location, duration, intensity, and etiology
31. hyperalgesia, allodynia, hyperpathia, and dysesthesia
32. transduction, transmission, perception, and modulation
33. ethnic and cultural values, developmental stage, environment and support people, previous pain experiences, and the meaning of the current pain
34. body, mind, spirit, and social relationships
35. (a) a pain history to obtain facts from the client and (b) direct observation of behaviors, physical signs of tissue damage, and secondary physiologic responses of the client
36. include pain location, intensity, quality, patterns, precipitating factors, alleviating factors, associated symptoms, effect on ADLs, past pain experiences, meaning of the pain to the person, coping resources, and affective responses
37. stop activity, tense muscles, and withdraw from the pain-provoking activities
38. distracting activities, relaxation techniques, imagery, meditation, biofeedback, hypnosis, cognitive-reframing, emotional counseling, and spiritually directed approaches such as therapeutic touch or Reiki
39. (1) This is called phantom pain, but it is a very real pain that needs to be treated. (2) With chronic pain, medication taken on a regular basis is often not strong enough to control the pain. (3) Morphine is probably the drug that provides him with relief, but sometimes exercising the leg can also be beneficial. (4) Since he needs the morphine he could be prescribed a supply to use at home when he has this extreme pain.
40. c. *Rationale:* Pain is the fifth vital sign and should be checked with the other vital signs. If the client is

grimacing or complaining of pain, it's already too late to get it under control. Vital signs are usually checked every four hours, so eight hours is too long to evaluate pain.

41. c. *Rationale:* Referred pain is the correct answer. Pain from the gallbladder can also mimic a heart attack. Chronic and acute pain is either continuous or comes and goes. Visceral pain is pain in an organ that radiates to hollow viscera.

42. b. *Rationale:* Somatic pain is a subcategory of physiologic pain. The other answers are other forms of pain.

43. d. *Rationale:* Nerves may be abnormal due to illness, injury, or undetermined reasons, causing pain.

44. c. *Rationale:* Neuropathic pain is a chronic type of pain that can be very hard to manage and difficult to treat. Research findings have pointed to inadequate treatment during the perioperative period as the potential cause of the client's continuing pain.

45. c. *Rationale:* Pain tolerance varies considerably from person to person, even within the same person at different times and in different circumstances.

46. b. *Rationale:* The client is always right. He is the only one who knows how much pain he is in and how much he can tolerate. It's good to make sure that the client understands the rating system, but do not judge clients by how they act. He may have been putting on a brave act for his visitors. Do not give a weaker medication unless you discuss it with the client.

47. d. *Rationale:* This is the most accurate answer. The others also have a degree of correctness but do not go far enough.

48. a. *Rationale:* This is the best answer, but all of these answers contribute to the way culture looks at and accepts pain.

49. d. *Rationale:* Although asking the client and using the scales are helpful, observing what activities the client does is often a better indicator of how the client really feels.

50. b. *Rationale:* Infants will behave differently to pain. Some have a higher tolerance than others. Some mothers can determine what is wrong from the infant's cry, but observing behavior might give a clue to where the pain is such as pulling on ears or pulling the legs up.

51. a. *Rationale:* When a person knows that someone cares, the person does not dwell on the pain.

52. a. *Rationale:* 100 mg IV = 300 mg po of morphine.

53. d. *Rationale:* Examples of coanalgesics that relieve pain are antidepressants, anticonvulsants, and local anesthetics.

54. d. *Rationale:* The use of placebos is frowned on. A placebo effect gives clients a feeling of relief. These are often sugar pills or even vitamins that are given to hypochondriac clients that have no need for drugs.

55. b. *Rationale:* These procedures may give some relief for short periods or may be long term, but the nerve endings can grow back and the pain will also return.

Chapter 19

1. l 2. o 3. k 4. p 5. m 6. h
7. a 8. c 9. i 10. s 11. t 12. r
13. e 14. g 15. d 16. x 17. j 18. z
19. v 20. n 21. y 22. q 23. b 24. w
25. u 26. f

27. water, soil, body surfaces such as the skin, and the intestinal tract
28. medical and surgical
29. bacteria, viruses, fungi, and parasites
30. through air, water, food, soil, body tissues and fluids, and inanimate objects
31. the urinary tract, the respiratory tract, bloodstream, and wounds
32. the etiologic agent, or microorganism; the place where the organism naturally resides (reservoir); a portal of exit from the reservoir; a method (mode) of transmission; a portal of entry into a host; and the susceptibility of the host
33. other humans, the client's own microorganisms, plants, animals, or the general environment
34. direct, indirect, airborne
35. sneezing, coughing, spitting, singing, or talking
36. age; clients receiving immune suppression treatment for cancer, for chronic illness, or following a successful organ transplant; and those with immune deficiency conditions
37. pain, swelling, redness, heat, and impaired function of the part
38. existing disease process, history of recurrent infections, current medications and therapeutic measures, current emotional stressors, nutritional status, and history of immunizations
39. decreases anti-inflammatory responses, depletes energy stores, leads to a state of exhaustion, and decreases resistance to infection
40. preventing infection, diagnosing and treating infection effectively, using antimicrobials wisely, and preventing transmission
41. maintain or restore defenses, avoid the spread of infectious organisms, reduce or alleviate problems associated with the infection
42. (1) Anyone entering the room should be gowned and gloved and should use the alcohol sanitizer before putting gloves on and after removing them and then wash hands. (2) Intubation done during surgery is through the mouth, and the client would have fewer problems with a tracheostomy. It will be easier to wean her from the respirator. (3) The sources of infection could be both the catheter and the tracheostomy. The nurse should observe the wound for signs of infection. (4) VRE is not curable but cultures will be negative with treatment.

43. b. *Rationale:* The World Health Organization is international. The CDC is for the United States,

OSHA deals with safety, and JCAHO deals with accrediting hospitals.

44. b. *Rationale:* The unfortunate problem is the longer a client remains in a hospital the higher the chances are of acquiring an infection. The old name was nosocomial infections. VRE and MRSA are both issues the medical profession is dealing with because of the overuse of antibiotics. We no longer have a strong antibiotic that will destroy resistant bacteria.
45. c. *Rationale:* Microorganisms may grow and multiply but do not cause disease. They create problems when moving from one area to another and can cause infections.
46. b. *Rationale:* The skin covers all of the body and keeps bacteria and viruses out as long as it is intact. The other answers are also part of the protection.
47. c. *Rationale:* Insipidus deals with the kidney's inability to concentrate urine. Mellitus is caused when the pancreas does not produce enough insulin and sugar damages the vascular system.
48. a. *Rationale:* This is the most complete answer. Three times a day may be good for brushing teeth, but hand washing is done too numerous to count. You should maintain hand hygiene when moving from dirty to clean areas.
49. c. *Rationale:* Sterile fields must be above the waist and protected from movement. Once it is left, it is no longer sterile. Option a is totally wrong, and option b could increase the likelihood of an infection to develop. Option d does not go as far as changing the dressing.
50. d. *Rationale:* Older adults may have all the normal signs listed in the other answers, but they may also become disoriented which is not a typical sign and usually is only seen in the elderly which is why infections can be missed.
51. b. *Rationale:* Nurses need to protect themselves and always report any splatters, especially blood, since many diseases can be spread through body fluids. Clients can only be tested if they give permission. Doing nothing or just cleaning up is not acceptable.
52. a. *Rationale:* Specific nursing activities are followed to interfere with the chain of infection, to prevent and control transmission of infectious organisms, and to promote care of the infected client.
53. c. *Rationale:* All of these answers can be effective, but nurses need to follow the procedures and policies established by the facility that employs them.
54. d. *Rationale:* Hand washing has been proven to be the number one measure against spreading infections. Hospitals now have sanitizers on all units and even by elevators so that visitors and staff can constantly destroy the microorganisms on their hands to prevent them from passing them on.
55. b. *Rationale:* Usually a person's natural defenses ward off the development of an infection. The normal flora, unless disrupted, will help protect from developing an infection or from being susceptible.
56. c. *Rationale:* The body constantly needs to rebuild and repair itself. Staying healthy will help to fight off infections through eating a nutritious diet.
57. a. *Rationale:* It destroys bacteria and can be found as properties in both antiseptics and disinfectants. Policies are made as to how strong it needs to be and how long it must be exposed to an area or equipment in order to be effective.

Chapter 20

1. f
2. p
3. o
4. q
5. s
6. a
7. r
8. l
9. v
10. e
11. u
12. z
13. x
14. w
15. t
16. c
17. j
18. g
19. d
20. y
21. m
22. n
23. i
24. k
25. h
26. b
27. sodium, potassium, chloride, and bicarbonate ions
28. urea and creatinine
29. radial, brachial, or femoral arteries
30. red meat; raw vegetables or fruits, particularly radishes, turnips, horseradish, and melons; or certain medications such as aspirin or nonsteroidal anti-inflammatory drugs, steroids, iron preparations, and anticoagulants
31. specific gravity, pH, glucose, ketones, protein, and occult blood
32. brain, spine, limbs and joints, heart, blood vessels, abdomen, and pelvis
33. injury, infection, or other pathology
34. sternum, iliac crests, anterior or posterior iliac spines, and proximal tibia in children
35. pretest phase, intratest phase, posttest phase
36. providing client comfort, privacy, and safety; explaining the purpose of a procedure for the specimen collection; using the correct procedure for obtaining the specimen; noting relevant information on the laboratory requisition slip; transporting the specimen promptly; and reporting abnormal findings
37. the bladder, ureteral orifices, and urethra
38. hemoglobin and hematocrit measurements, erythrocyte (RBC) count, leukocyte (WBC) count, red blood cell (RBC) indices, and may also include a differential white cell count
39. (1) A 24-hour urine test is usually started in the morning after the first void of the day. (2) Hematocrit and hemoglobin tests will show if the bleeding continues or has stopped related to the red blood cell count. (3) A positive Hemoccult would indicate that she is bleeding in the gastrointestinal system. (4) The nurse needs to explain the tests to the client and assist her in completing the collection of urine and feces.
40. c. *Rationale:* Blood tests are the most common tests. The other tests are used to diagnose specific problems.

41. a. *Rationale:* Urea is the end product of protein metabolism. BUN is blood urea nitrogen.
42. d. *Rationale:* The glycosylated test shows the hyperglycemia for three to four months. Chemstrip and glucometer are used to test a current reading. A_{c1} should be A_{1c}, which is another name for glycosylated hemoglobin.
43. b. *Rationale:* A Hemoccult is done to check for blood in feces. Peroxidase is an enzyme used in the reagent so that it shows if blood is present. Guaiac is another word for feces. Reagent is a substance used in a chemical reaction to detect a specific substance.
44. c. *Rationale:* MRI and CAT are used to visualize anatomic structures. LP is a lumbar puncture that removes cerebrospinal fluid for examination.
45. d. *Rationale:* A paracentesis is done to remove the ascites or the fluid in the abdominal cavity. LP removes cerebrospinal fluid. PET creates images with an isotope.
46. b. *Rationale:* Chemotherapeutic drugs can be instilled through a thoracentesis. A biopsy cannot be performed by doing a thoracentesis. A culture and sensitivity could be performed on the fluid withdrawn, but that does not answer the question.
47. a. *Rationale:* White blood cells attack foreign bodies that enter the body. They increase with bacteria to fight them off and decrease with viruses. Option b is backwards, c is not an answer to the question, and d is why a WBC is checked.
48. b. *Rationale:* This is the correct answer for the normal specific gravity of urine.
49. a. *Rationale:* The nurse compares the previous and current test results and modifies nursing interventions as needed during the postphase. Intratest focuses on specimen collection. The major focus of the pretest phase is client preparation.
50. c. *Rationale:* Arterial stick is used for blood gases, a phlebotomist performs venipuncture, and a finger stick is used for a glucose test or with capillary tubes.
51. d. *Rationale:* Anemia is caused by blood loss, especially the RBCs that have the heme needed to carry oxygen. Polycythemia is higher RBCs than normal counts, hypervolemia is an increase in fluid volume, and hemodilution results from the hypervolemia.
52. b. *Rationale:* The CBC is a basic screening test and one of the most frequently ordered blood tests. RBCs, H & H, and WBCs are included in the CBC.
53. d. *Rationale:* Urea and creatinine are metabolically produced substances and are routinely used to evaluate renal function. Nitrogen is also a waste product of protein and bilirubin.
54. c. *Rationale:* The peak level indicates the highest concentration of the drug, and the trough level represents the lowest concentration. They are used to check the therapeutic level of the drug. This is often done with antibiotics that are given intravenously.

Chapter 21

1. f 2. d 3. e 4. b 5. g 6. c
7. a
8. motor vehicle accidents, falls, drowning, fire and burns, poisoning, inhalation and ingestion of foreign objects, and use of firearms
9. unsafe work environments, residence in neighborhoods with high crime rates, access to guns and ammunition, insufficient income to buy safety equipment or make necessary repairs, and access to illicit drugs
10. age, development, lifestyle, mobility, health status, sensory-perceptual alterations, emotional states, ability to communicate, safety awareness, and environmental factors
11. machinery, industrial belts and pulleys, and chemicals
12. worker fatigue, noise, air pollution, working at great heights, working in subterranean areas
13. adequate street lighting, safe water, safe sewage treatment, and regulation of sanitation in food buying
14. excess noise, crime, traffic congestion, dilapidated housing, or unprotected creeks and landfills
15. medication errors, wrong-site surgery, restraint-related injuries or death, falls, burns, pressure ulcers, or mistaken identity
16. limited short-term memory, being late or in a hurry, limited ability to multitask, interruptions, stress, fatigue and other physiologic factors, environmental factors
17. noting pertinent indicators in the nursing history and physical examination, using specifically developed risk assessment tools, and evaluating the client's environment
18. olfactory, visual, tactile, taste, or other sensory impairments
19. anthrax, botulism, plague, viral hemorrhagic fevers, smallpox, and tularemia
20. critical access hospitals, long-term care facilities, or home care agencies
21. risk for poisoning, risk for suffocation, risk for trauma, latex allergy response, risk for latex allergy response, contamination, risk for contamination, risk for aspiration, risk for disuse syndrome
22. White men are the most likely to commit suicide. Uncontrollable pain, loss of a loved one, and major life changes can be contributing factors. Major depression and social isolation increase the risk of suicide. Older adults rarely threaten to commit suicide; they just do it.
23. (1) Clients with dementia need to be monitored 24 hours a day, and the facility would normally be the safest way to go. (2) Dementia clients are often not as aware of safety issues and do not think about what they should do to remain safe, so they are often more prone to physical injuries. (3) Many long-term facilities use a beeper system that has an alarm placed on a wheelchair or on the bed to protect the clients by alarming if they should try to get up. Another method

is to have low beds with pads on the floor so the client that falls out of bed will not be harmed. (4) It is unfortunate that an injury occurred, and ultimately the staff is at fault. He should have been evaluated for potential injuries, and steps should have been instituted to keep him safe.

24. d. *Rationale:* Medical errors unfortunately cause more deaths than all the others.
25. b. *Rationale:* Between 44,000 and 98,000 people die in the United States each year due to medical errors in hospitals. These deaths are not necessary if medical personnel think about what they are doing and if the equipment used on clients is safe and working appropriately. Safety starts with nurses doing their job to the best of their ability and within the scope of practice for their licensing. The majority of the errors could have been avoided if better systems of care were in place.
26. a. *Rationale:* This tool directs the nurse to appraise the factors affecting safety.
27. b. *Rationale:* Suicides by firearms, drugs, and automobile exhaust gases are the most common. These are often caused by economic deprivation, family breakup, and the availability of firearms.
28. d. *Rationale:* Although these answers are all correct and are steps that should be taken to prevent the problems, the first thing that needs to be done is to identify youth that are at risk.
29. b. *Rationale:* In the past, the question was always: Who caused the problem? Now the focus is to prevent errors. In order to do that, finding out how it happened and how to prevent it from happening again is more important.
30. c. *Rationale:* Older adults are committing suicide at an increased rate and usually succeed because they actually want to die. The other answers can be part of the total answer since they have lived longer and have more knowledge as how to accomplish it.
31. b. *Rationale:* Restraints should be used only in extreme situations and the client has to be constantly observed. The restraints need to be removed every hour to check the skin, offer the client food and beverage, and meet the client's needs. In some instances, such as the ICU, restraints are used to protect the client from pulling out central lines, IVs, and ventilator tubes or any other tubes that if removed could harm the client.
32. b. *Rationale:* This is the best answer but the other answers also create problems for client safety. Ratios need to be regulated and hours for nurses need to be limited so that nurses will not get burned out and act in an unsafe manner.
33. a. *Rationale:* These answers have all contributed to nurses being available for disasters and being alert for more than usual cases of germs that could be from germ warfare.
34. b. *Rationale:* Young children have a habit of biting window sills and putting things in their mouths that are not edible. Paint used in houses built prior to 1978 contains lead. Federal money has been granted to lead-proof older homes to protect children from lead poisoning that causes brain damage.
35. c. *Rationale:* Teenagers go through many changes in a short period of time. Each new adventure helps to build on skills they will need to get through life, and sports activities will develop teamwork and conflict resolution.
36. d. *Rationale:* When children are abused they can carry that over in their adult years because they have learned the behavior as normal. This cycle will continue until someone is able to break it.
37. c. *Rationale:* Falls are the leading cause of injuries among older adults and infants.
38. a. *Rationale:* Seizures last for short periods, and nurses need to observe in order to be able to document and report the incident to a physician. The client needs to be protected from falls. If they are in bed with the top rails up, they are usually protected from injuries. It is important for nurses to have good observation skills.
39. b. *Rationale:* Clients who suffocate lose oxygen in the brain if breathing is not restored, resulting in cardiac arrest and death.

Chapter 22

1. e 2. l 3. m 4. q 5. r 6. i
7. k 8. p 9. o 10. n 11. a 12. d
13. f 14. c 15. s 16. h 17. g 18. j
19. b
20. care of the skin, hair, nails, teeth, oral and nasal cavities, eyes, ears, and perineal-genital areas
21. protects underlying tissues from injury by preventing the passage of microorganisms, regulates the body temperature, secretes sebum, transmits sensations through nerve receptors, and produces and absorbs vitamin D
22. water, sodium, potassium, chloride, glucose, urea, and lactate
23. a nursing health history to determine the client's skin care practices, self-care abilities, and past or current skin problems; physical assessment of the skin; and identification of clients at risk for developing skin impairments
24. client's balance, ability to sit unsupported, activity tolerance, coordination, adequate muscle strength, appropriate joint range of motion, vision, and the client's preferences
25. normal nail and foot care practices, type of footwear worn, self-care abilities, presence of risk factors for foot problems, any foot discomfort, and any perceived problems with foot mobility
26. calluses, corns, unpleasant odors, plantar warts, fissures between the toes, and fungal infections
27. bacteria, molecules of saliva, and remnants of epithelial cells and leukocytes
28. lack of knowledge and the inability to maintain oral hygiene

29. inadequate nutrition, lack of money and/or insurance for dental care, excessive intake of refined sugars, and family history of periodontal disease
30. poor fluid intake, heavy smoking, alcohol use, high salt intake, anxiety, and many medications
31. antiviral, antibacterial, and antifungal
32. dandruff, hair loss, ticks, pediculosis, and scabies
33. the person habitually scratches, there are scratches on the skin, and there are hemorrhagic spots on the skin where the lice have sucked blood
34. stimulates the circulation of blood in the scalp, distributes the oil along the hair shaft, and helps to arrange the hair.
35. They cannot be seen and thus have cosmetic value, they are highly effective in correcting some astigmatisms, they are safer than glasses for some physical activities, they do not fog as eyeglasses do, and they provide better vision in many cases.
36. (1) Most likely this would be lice although there are also outbreaks of bedbugs, especially in hotels. (2) Treatment includes washing all linens and clothing and treating all family members. (3) If it is lice, they will spread from child to child. All students that were around or in contact should be checked and treated if lice or eggs are found. (4) If the hotel is the source, it should be reported to the health department and to the management so they can rectify the problem.
37. b. *Rationale:* Although these are all problems, unfortunately, Alzheimer's is the most prevalent and can also start at an earlier age.
38. c. *Rationale:* Tight shoes cause friction and pressure, restricting circulation on a bony prominence. A corn can be removed. If shoes are not tight in the toe box, it should not return.
39. c. *Rationale:* Placing an infant in bed with a bottle is not good for the teeth. The solutions cause demineralization of the tooth enamel and promote decay.
40. a. *Rationale:* Plaque forms tartar and then leads to tooth decay and especially problems with the gums, which can promote a loss of teeth.
41. c. *Rationale:* Nurses and UAPs need to promote oral hygiene and learn how to properly care for another's teeth. Dementia can limit clients' abilities to care for their dental needs, and physical limitations may also be a factor.
42. c. *Rationale:* About 35% of older adults in the community have cerumen impaction in one or both ears. They often use cotton swabs that only push the wax in further and impairs the hearing.
43. a. *Rationale:* Eyes should be cleaned away from the lacrimal duct so it does not become occluded. The other answers would cause significant problems.
44. c. *Rationale:* Eyes that cannot provide lacrimal fluid to wash the eyes need to be kept moist with eye drops to prevent eye damage.
45. d. *Rationale:* Hearing aids are used by all ages of clients and help to convert sound to electric energy to improve hearing.
46. c. *Rationale:* Hearing aids used in the ear canal are less visible and do not interfere with telephone use or the wearing of eyeglasses.
47. c. *Rationale:* Nurses need to care for the client and it is easier if the bed is not wide.
48. b. *Rationale:* Side rails are not used for safety measures since most clients can crawl over them and injure themselves. The safest way to use them is as a client helper.
49. c. *Rationale:* Bed cradles are used for burn victims so the sheets do not dry on the skin and pull it off. They can also be used for clients that have lupus where touching the skin is painful.
50. c. *Rationale:* This is the best answer, although now many hospitals use fitted sheets and only the top sheet and blanket have to be mitered.
51. a. *Rationale:* Making a bed allows the nurse time to observe the client and to assess the skin for breakdowns and any drainage from wounds. Time with clients should always be used productively.

Chapter 23

1. h 2. k 3. z 4. o 5. n 6. j
7. y 8. x 9. s 10. f 11. b 12. t
13. d 14. p 15. u 16. w 17. m 18. l
19. v 20. c 21. i 22. q 23. a 24. e
25. r 26. g

27. generic name, official name, chemical name, and trademark or brand name
28. according to their source, physical and chemical properties, tests for purity and identity, method of storage, assay, category, and normal dosages
29. agonist and antagonist
30. know how nursing practice acts in their areas define and limit their functions, and be able to recognize the limits of their own knowledge and skill
31. a double-locked drawer, cupboard, medication cart, or computer-controlled dispensing system
32. the name of the client, the date and time of administration, the name of the drug, the dosage, and the signature of the person who prepared and gave the drug
33. opiates, barbiturates, ethyl alcohol, and tobacco
34. biliary obstruction, renal damage, and malformations of the fetus
35. laxatives, antacids, vitamins, headache remedies, and cough and cold medications
36. drugs unavailable for purchase under any circumstances, such as heroin (in the United States); and drugs normally available with a prescription that are being obtained through illegal channels
37. full name of the client, date and time the order is written, name of the drug to be administered, dosage

of the drug, frequency of administration, route of administration, and signature of the person writing the order
38. needles, dental wires, surgical blades, broken glass, lancets, broken capillary pipettes
39. gender, size, body composition
40. drug metabolism and variations in enzymes
41. right medication, dose, time, route, client, client education, documentation, to refuse, assessment, evaluation
42. include unpleasant taste of the drugs, irritation of the gastric mucosa, irregular absorption from the gastrointestinal tract, slow absorption, and may harm the client's teeth
43. liver, kidneys, and brain
44. (1) The abbreviations are standard and would be recognized by all nurses. (2) Other orders may be for a diet, possibly an antibiotic, oximeter checks, respiratory treatments, culture and sensitivity for the sputum, and lab work such as a CBC to check white cell count and a chem 7 to check her electrolytes. (3) A possible diagnosis could be pneumonia or bronchitis. (4) A question that needs to be asked is does she smoke and how much, and also if there is a history of asthma and any drug allergies.
45. d. *Rationale:* Both the physician and the nurse are at fault. Any order that is not safe or a drug that should not be given should be questioned and double-checked with both the physician ordering the drug and the pharmacist who dispenses it.
46. b. *Rationale:* Varying degrees of psychologic dependence range from mild desire to craving and compulsive use of the drug.
47. b. *Rationale:* The formulary is the only book that lists therapeutic values. These books are all valuable for nurses to have a better understanding of drugs.
48. c. *Rationale:* A severe allergic reaction causes early symptoms that are subjective, such as swelling in the mouth and tongue, acute shortness of breath, acute hypotension, and tachycardia.
49. c. *Rationale:* Food can combine with molecules of certain drugs and change the molecular structure, subsequently inhibiting or preventing their absorption.
50. b. *Rationale:* The highly vascular nature of muscle tissue promotes absorption with increased blood flow.
51. b. *Rationale:* These answers are all variations on the same theme with words switched around to make sure you read questions carefully. Option b is the only correctly written answer.
52. b. *Rationale:* Research has shown that certain medications may work well at usual therapeutic dosages for certain ethnic groups but be toxic for others. This opens a new field of awareness for nurses when caring for clients and dispensing medications. It shows one dose does not fit all.
53. d. *Rationale:* They are eliminated by the kidneys in the urine, but some are also excreted in the feces.
54. d. *Rationale:* All medications are dispensed in the metric system. An example would be aspirin, which is dispensed in 81 mg and 325 mg. Although the average person does not know what this means, it is important for the nurse to have a good understanding to calculate safe dosages.
55. d. *Rationale:* Although social services could help, usually it is only a one-time help. Providing medications on discharge also does not solve the problem long term, but resources may be available where free meds can be received directly from the manufacturer for as long as the problem exists.
56. c. *Rationale:* The goal is providing correct medications to the patient at all transition points within the hospital. Most medical errors are caused when clients are transferred.
57. a. *Rationale:* In an attempt to limit medication errors from happening, JCAHO requires at least two identifiers to be certain the right drug gets to the right client.
58. c. *Rationale:* With all clients, especially children, nurses need to gain and maintain their trust. The only way is through honesty.
59. a. *Rationale:* Older adults have a slower metabolism and may need smaller amounts of drugs as they age. Diet, activities, and other medications taken all play a role in how much should be prescribed.
60. b. *Rationale:* Medications given as injections need to be handled carefully. If a medication is given to the wrong client or the wrong dose is given, counteractive measures must be immediate.

Chapter 24

1. h 2. k 3. l 4. q 5. z 6. n
7. r 8. o 9. s 10. c 11. p 12. i
13. a 14. e 15. j 16. u 17. t 18. v
19. x 20. w 21. y 22. m 23. b 24. g
25. f 26. d

27. genetics, age, and the underlying health of the individual,
28. clean wounds, clean-contaminated wounds, contaminated wounds, dirty or infected wounds
29. immobility and inactivity, inadequate nutrition, fecal and urinary incontinence, decreased mental status, diminished sensation, excessive body heat, advanced age, and the presence of certain chronic conditions
30. weight loss, muscle atrophy, and the loss of subcutaneous tissue
31. protein, carbohydrates, fluids, zinc, and vitamin C
32. digestive enzymes in feces, gastric tube drainage, and urea in urine
33. loss of lean body mass, generalized thinning of the epidermis, decreased strength and elasticity of the skin due to changes in the collagen fibers of the dermis, increased dryness due to a decrease in the amount of oil produced by the sebaceous glands, diminished pain

perception due to a reduction in the number of cutaneous end organs responsible for the sensation of pressure and light touch, diminished venous and arterial flow due to aging vascular walls

34. sensory perception, moisture, activity, mobility, nutrition, and friction and shear
35. general physical condition, mental state, activity, mobility, and incontinence
36. the type of healing, the location and size of the wound, and the health of the client
37. inflammatory, proliferative, and maturation or remodeling
38. hemostasis and phagocytosis
39. serous, purulent, and sanguineous
40. tinges of blue, green, or yellow
41. age, nutritional status, lifestyle, and medications
42. protein, carbohydrates, lipids, vitamins A and C, and minerals iron, zinc, and copper
43. rapid thready pulse, cold clammy skin, pallor, lowered blood pressure
44. antibiotics, irrigation, surgical incision to open and drain the tract, or vacuum therapy for large tracts
45. location of the ulcer, related to a bony prominence, size of ulcer in centimeters, presence of undermining or sinus tracts, stage of the ulcer, color of the wound bed and location of necrosis or eschar, condition of the wound margins, integrity of surrounding skin, clinical signs of infection
46. supporting wound healing, preventing pressure ulcers, treating pressure ulcers, dressing and cleaning wounds, applying heat and cold, and supporting and immobilizing wounds
47. maintaining moist wound healing, providing sufficient nutrition and hydration, preventing wound infections, and proper positioning
48. prone, supine, right and left lateral (side-lying), and right and left Sims' positions
49. gentle cleansing; protecting periwound skin with alcohol-free barrier film; filling dead space with hydrogel or alginate; covering with an appropriate dressing such as transparent film, hydrocolloid dressing, or a clear absorbent acrylic dressing; and changing the dressing as infrequently as possible
50. sharp, mechanical, chemical, and autolytic
51. to protect the wound from mechanical injury, to protect the wound from microbial contamination, to provide or maintain moist wound healing, to provide thermal insulation, to absorb drainage or debride a wound or both, to prevent a hemorrhage, to splint or immobilize the wound site and thereby facilitate healing and prevent injury
52. the location, size, and type of the wound; the amount of exudate; whether the wound requires debridement or is infected; and such considerations as frequency of dressing change, ease or difficulty of dressing application, and cost
53. (1) The burns will allow for the introduction of microorganisms that can cause an infection. Burns weep, which will cause loss of fluid that will need to be replaced. (2) Although he is on bed rest with traction, he will need to be turned and positioned and his body will need to be checked often to make sure no breakdowns occur. (3) He will need to have his temperature and other vitals monitored, but also his pain level. He should be kept comfortable so he can rest and allow the body to heal. (4) As eschar forms, it will need to be removed from each area to promote new skin growth.
54. b. *Rationale:* The skin protects all the other organs and helps to maintain health and protect the individual from injury.
55. d. *Rationale:* These answers are all important for nurses, but they need to know that intact skin promotes better health. Intact skin refers to the presence of normal skin and skin layers uninterrupted by wounds.
56. d. *Rationale:* All of these things happen when tissues do not receive nutrients, but the end result is a breakdown especially over bony prominences.
57. a. *Rationale:* Sliding a client in bed causes friction and pressure to the coccyx areas and can tear the skin, allowing bacteria to enter. These areas can become deep and large if left untreated, damaging the blood vessels and tissues.
58. a. *Rationale:* When diseases compromise the delivery of oxygen to tissues, the ability to maintain health becomes more difficult.
59. c. *Rationale:* This occurs where the tissue surfaces have been approximated with minimal tissue loss. These wounds heal the best and scarring is minimal.
60. d. *Rationale:* Scabs are made up of dead cells, clots, and dying tissue. This helps to keep out microorganisms from invading and causing an infection.
61. d. *Rationale:* This method allows the body's own enzymes in the drainage to break down the necrotic tissue. This takes longer.
62. a. *Rationale:* Maggots secrete enzymes that break down necrotic tissue, leaving healthy tissue alone. They eat bacteria and decrease bacterial growth through the rise in surface pH that results from their presence.
63. a. *Rationale:* This promotes epithelial growth, hastens healing, and reduces the risk of infection.
64. c. *Rationale:* These straps prevent skin irritation and discomfort caused by removing the adhesive each time the dressing is changed. They can hold larger dressings to prevent drainage from getting on the skin or clothing.
65. c. *Rationale:* Infections can have increased amounts of purulent drainage and it needs to be removed so healthy tissue will granulate. Suctioning out the drainage keeps the wound drier.

66. b. *Rationale:* Using heat can cause fainting if the blood pressure drops. Clients with cardiac or pulmonary problems will be affected by the vasodilation.
67. a. *Rationale:* Heat or cold should be removed after 20 minutes to prevent the rebound effect and to protect the client from serious problems.
68. d. *Rationale:* Dead white blood cells from phagocytosis form purulent drainage found in infected wounds.

Chapter 25

1. g 2. i 3. r 4. l 5. j 6. q
7. a 8. m 9. e 10. p 11. h 12. u
13. o 14. d 15. t 16. n 17. f 18. c
19. b 20. s 21. k

22. preoperative, intraoperative, and postoperative
23. include assessing the client, identifying potential or actual health problems, planning specific care based on the individual's needs, and providing preoperative teaching for the client, the family, and significant others
24. hospital-based inpatient and outpatient surgical/laser/endoscopy suites, physician office-based surgical suites (outpatient), and/or freestanding outpatient/ambulatory surgical centers
25. purpose, degree of urgency, and degree of risk
26. client's age, general health, nutritional status, use of medications, and mental status
27. a chronic disease, such as cardiovascular disease, chronic lung disease, or diabetes
28. obesity and malnutrition
29. delayed wound healing, wound infection, and fluid and electrolyte alterations
30. anticoagulants, tranquilizers, corticosteroids, diuretics
31. the nature of and the reason for the surgery, all available options and the risks associated with each option, the risks of the surgical procedure and its potential outcomes, name and qualifications of the surgeon performing the procedure, the right to refuse consent or later withdraw consent
32. the consumption of clear liquids up to two hours before elective surgery requiring general anesthesia, regional anesthesia, or sedation-analgesia; a light breakfast (e.g., tea and toast) six hours before the procedure; a heavier meal eight hours before surgery
33. secobarbital and diazepam, morphine and meperidine, atropine, scopolamine and glycopyrrolate, cimetidine and ranitidine, Innovar
34. verify the client at the time surgery is scheduled, during admission, and whenever the client is transferred to another caregiver; mark the operative site in an unambiguous manner; take a time-out before surgery to conduct a final verification of the correct client, procedure, and site
35. blocking awareness centers in the brain so that amnesia (loss of memory), analgesia (insensibility to pain), hypnosis (artificial sleep), and relaxation (rendering a part of the body less tense) occur
36. intravenous infusion or by inhalation of gases through a mask or through an endotracheal tube inserted into the trachea
37. the client's vital signs, ECG, oxygen saturation, fluid intake and urinary output, estimate of blood loss, arterial and venous pressures, pulmonary artery pressures, and laboratory values such as blood glucose, hemoglobin, hematocrit, serum electrolytes, and arterial blood gases
38. position the client appropriately for surgery; perform preoperative skin preparation; assist in preparing and maintaining the sterile field; open and dispense sterile supplies during surgery; provide medications and solutions for the sterile field; monitor and maintain a safe, aseptic environment; manage catheters, tubes, drains, and specimens; perform sponge, sharp, and instrument counts; document nursing care provided and the client's response to interventions
39. includes assessment, diagnosis, outcome identification, planning, implementation, and evaluation
40. pallor, perspiration, muscle tension, and reluctance to cough, move, or ambulate
41. pain management, appropriate positioning, incentive spirometry and deep-breathing and coughing exercises, leg exercises, early ambulation, adequate hydration, diet, promoting urinary and bowel elimination, suction maintenance, and wound care
42. appearance, size, drainage, swelling, pain, and the status of a drain or tubes
43. (1) Operating rooms need to be sterile to protect the clients from microorganisms that could cause infections. (2) Student nurses are usually versed in the procedures of the OR and would not have entered a sterile room without another nurse. (3) The student needs to tell the nurse about the instrument, but since it was not placed back on the sterile field it would probably not be used. (4) The student should have probably left it on the floor so there would not be a mistake in using it.
44. c. *Rationale:* A child's developmental level and age-appropriate communication are important in implementing the pediatric plan of care and being able to explain the procedure and what to expect when it is finished.
45. c. *Rationale:* A physician is responsible to inform a client about the procedure and all the risks that are involved. Clients also need to ask questions and fully understand their responsibility in helping to regain their health.
46. c. *Rationale:* The nurse is responsible for the paperwork, but any further explanations need to be handled by the surgeon.
47. a. *Rationale:* Surgery affects the body in many ways. The client needs to be prepared and go into surgery with a good understanding of the procedure in order to be confident about the outcome.

48. c. *Rationale:* All clients should be started on discharge planning the minute they are admitted to the hospital.
49. b. *Rationale:* The skin has normal flora that protects the client, but if allowed to enter a wound it could cause an infection. It is imperative to have the client shower prior to surgery.
50. a. *Rationale:* The circulating nurse and scrub person are responsible for accounting of all sponges, needles, and instruments at the close of surgery.
51. a. *Rationale:* Having any invasive procedure changes the dynamics of the body. When cutting open any area, it starts the WBCs to start the healing process and to fight off potential infections. This is only one aspect that occurs. Disruptions will depend on the extent of surgery and the location.
52. a. *Rationale:* Keeping the client in good alignment protects the muscles from injury.
53. c. *Rationale:* This is the best answer. Surgical procedures require drugs that alter thought processes. Nurses need to monitor clients until the anesthesia is out of their system and they can function again.
54. a. *Rationale:* This position keeps the drainage from going down the respiratory tree.
55. b. *Rationale:* The pressure of an arm against the chest reduces chest expansion. The client needs to fully expand to prevent postop complications.
56. c. *Rationale:* The client's fluid loss during surgery needs to be replaced to maintain adequate I & O and keep the blood pressure up.
57. d. *Rationale:* Clients are instructed on coughing and deep breathing. By using the incentive spirometer, they will prevent the lungs from collapsing from a buildup of mucus.
58. d. *Rationale:* Clients need to be moved every two hours. If able, they should ambulate. If that is contraindicated, sitting would help them to expand their lungs.
59. b. *Rationale:* Exudates interfere with the formation of granulation tissue so suctioning a wound will allow for the incision to heal faster.

Chapter 26

1. e   2. i   3. j   4. g   5. l   6. a
7. h   8. f   9. c   10. k   11. d   12. b
13. growth, development, and survival
14. reception and perception
15. a stimulus, a receptor, impulse conduction, and perception
16. the reticular excitatory area (REA) and the reticular inhibitory area (RIA)
17. visual (sight), auditory (hearing), olfactory (smell), tactile (touch), and gustatory (taste)
18. kinesthetic or visceral; also gustatory is both external and internal
19. conscious thought, reality orientation, problem solving, judgment, and comprehension
20. pain, lack of sleep, and worry, increased quantity or quality of internal stimuli, such as pain, dyspnea, or anxiety; increased quantity or quality of external stimuli, such as a noisy health care setting, intrusive diagnostic studies, or contacts with many strangers; and inability to disregard stimuli selectively, perhaps as a result of nervous system disturbances or medications that stimulate the arousal mechanism
21. developmental stage, culture, level of stress, medications and illness, and lifestyle
22. aspirin, furosemide (Lasix), the aminoglycosides, and certain drugs given for cancer chemotherapy
23. nursing history, mental status examination, physical examination, identification of clients at risk, the client's environment, and social support network
24. inattention to others, recent mood swings, difficulty following clear instructions, frequent requests to have something repeated, and unusually loud radio or television volumes
25. visual acuity, using a Snellen chart or other reading material such as a newspaper, and visual fields; hearing acuity, by observing the client's conversation with others and by performing the whisper test and the Weber and Rinne tuning fork tests; olfactory sense, by identifying specific aromas; gustatory sense, by identifying three tastes such as lemon, salt, and sugar; tactile sense, by testing light touch, sharp and dull sensation, two-point discrimination, hot and cold sensation, vibration sense, position sense, and stereognosis
26. withdrawal from contact with others to avoid embarrassment or dependence on others, negative self-image, reports of lack of meaningful communication with others, and absence of opportunities to discuss fears or concerns that facilitate coping mechanisms
27. (1) Social services can always devise a plan for the client to return home with help or to help him get any special equipment he may need to function independently. (2) Nurses should do general assessments on cognitive reasoning and make sure he is able to care for himself. (3) With the information given and with help from his family, he should be able to be discharged to home. (4) Chronologic age does not always determine what a person is capable of doing. The nurse must assess his abilities and look at any potential issues where he may need help as he heals.
28. a. *Rationale:* Visceral organs may produce stimuli that make a person aware of them (e.g., a full stomach).
29. b. *Rationale:* When organs do not receive adequate blood flow, it decreases awareness and slows responses.
30. d. *Rationale:* Uncontrolled diabetes mellitus can impair vision and cause blindness. Often it is diagnosed late and damage has already been started.
31. d. *Rationale:* Sensory overload can prevent the brain from ignoring or responding to specific stimuli when too much stimulation is received at the same time.

32. b. *Rationale:* The normal should be 45 decibels. With all the equipment and nurses talking, it can be as high as 60–83, causing a sensory overload to the clients trying to rest.
33. a. *Rationale:* Discharge planning incorporates a reassessment of the client's abilities for self-care, the availability and skills of support people, financial resources, and the need for referrals and home health services.
34. c. *Rationale:* Any sexually transmitted infection should be checked and treated to protect the lives of the mother and the baby.
35. a. *Rationale:* When one sense is lost, other senses will become stronger to replace the lost sense.
36. b. *Rationale:* Listening carefully when visually impaired will help to analyze the message that is being relayed.
37. a. *Rationale:* Since all the other answers are the opposite of what they should be, this is the only correct answer.
38. d. *Rationale:* Nurses should not overstimulate their clients or scare them but should announce that they are there and what their intentions are.
39. d. *Rationale:* Although many things can be done to orient a confused client, the most important would be to see what the client knows and how oriented he or she is at a given moment.
40. c. *Rationale:* Clients need to be stimulated by talking to them. You never know what they can hear and understand, even in an unconscious state.

Chapter 27

1. c   2. f   3. h   4. k   5. j   6. l
7. o   8. g   9. m   10. a   11. e   12. b
13. n   14. i   15. d
16. how one thinks, talks, and acts; how one sees and treats another person; choices one makes; ability to give and receive love; ability to take action and to change things
17. self-knowledge, self-expectation, social self, social evaluation
18. beliefs, attitudes, motivations, strengths, and limitations
19. vocational performance, intellectual functioning, personal appearance and physical attractiveness, sexual attractiveness and performance, being liked by others, ability to cope with and resolve problems, independence, particular talents
20. personal identity, body image, role performance, and self-esteem
21. name, sex, age, race, ethnic origin or culture, occupation or roles, talents, and other situational characteristics
22. pain, pleasure, fatigue, and physical movement
23. certain personal standards, aspirations, goals, and values
24. ability to appraise one's own strengths, the desire to follow in the steps of role models, and the feedback received from colleagues and clients
25. beliefs, values, personality, and character
26. The infant learns that the physical self is separate and different from the environment. The child internalizes others' attitudes toward self. The child and adult internalize the standards of society.
27. integrated body image, role performance, and self-esteem into a complete self-concept
28. clothing, makeup, hairstyle, jewelry, and other things intimately connected to the person such as body prostheses, dentures, hairpieces, wheelchairs, canes, and eyeglasses
29. husband, parent, brother, son, employee, friend, nurse, and church member
30. support network, sufficient finances, and organizations
31. acceptance, denial, withdrawal, and depression
32. Create a quiet, private environment. Minimize interruptions if possible. Maintain appropriate eye contact. Sit at eye level with the client. Demonstrate an interest in the client's concerns. Indicate acceptance of the client by not criticizing, frowning, or demonstrating shock. Ask open-ended questions to encourage the client to talk rather than close-ended questions that tend to block free sharing. Avoid asking more personal questions than are actually needed. Minimize writing detailed notes during the interview because this can create client concern that confidential material is being "recorded" as well as interfere with your ability to focus on what the client is saying. Determine whether the family can provide additional information. Maintain confidentiality. Be aware of your own biases and discomforts that could influence the assessment. Consider how the client's behavior is influenced by culture.
33. (1) Reeja's self-concept would be negative and she would have a hard time maintaining interpersonal relationships. This could drop her resistance to psychologic and physical illnesses. (2) Even though it was not her fault, the failure would promote a low self-esteem and she would have negative feelings about the country and the people in this country. (3) Role strain would occur if she had an occupation in a mostly male profession, but nursing is mostly females. (4) Teaching cultural differences is new to nursing. These may have been older nurses who have a very low opinion of foreign trained nurses or they may have been worried about their own jobs. They may treat clients differently. At least in the new hospital she was treated better.
34. c. *Rationale:* We are not born with a self-concept. It forms and changes as we interact with others.
35. d. *Rationale:* Self-concept is an ongoing process. As we change and grow, our self-concept will continue to change and evolve.
36. b. *Rationale:* Only a great discrepancy can cause low self-esteem.

37. c. *Rationale:* Our values and life experiences help to develop who and what we are.
38. a. *Rationale:* A basic concept involves two steps: one from our viewpoint and one from others.
39. d. *Rationale:* Tension and a decrease in self-esteem leads to embarrassment.
40. a. *Rationale:* Young children spend more time with their families. The culture of the family influences all aspects of their lives. Later, their relationships with peers will influence them, but what they learned from the family will always stay with them.
41. c. *Rationale:* Nurses need to have a therapeutic relationship and help clients help themselves.
42. c. *Rationale:* Maintaining and evaluating one's self-concept is an ongoing process and can change with each new event.
43. a. *Rationale:* The individual sees himself or herself as a unique person.
44. c. *Rationale:* The cognitive is the knowledge of the material body. The affective includes the sensations of the body, such as pain, pleasure, fatigue, and physical movement.
45. c. *Rationale:* Adolescents see rock stars and movie stars as the ideal and try to follow their standards even though those are not realistic and not what they should be reaching for.

Chapter 28

1. g   2. p   3. k   4. a   5. j   6. r
7. s   8. q   9. e   10. c 11. n 12. o
13. u 14. t 15. w 16. y 17. x 18. d
19. v 20. b 21. h 22. l 23. m 24. f
25. i
26. physiologic, psychosocial, and cultural
27. tender breasts, water retention, and skin eruptions or pimples
28. bed rest, administration of analgesics, application of heat to the abdomen, certain exercises such as abdominal muscle strengthening, biofeedback, and nonsteroidal anti-inflammatory medications
29. about sex, sexual actions and their consequences, the individual's right to make a decision regarding ways to express oneself sexually, and the responsibilities of each person with respect to sexual activity
30. abstinence, pills, timed-release transdermal patches and implants, diaphragms, intrauterine devices, the rhythm method, and condoms
31. touching, hugging, romantic gestures, comfort, warmth, dressing up, joy, spirituality, and beauty
32. "the integration of the somatic, emotional, intellectual, and social aspects of sexual being, in ways that are positively enriching and that enhance personality, communication, and love"
33. sexual self-concept, body image, gender identity, gender-role behavior, and freedoms and responsibilities
34. pregnancy, aging, trauma, disease, and therapies
35. physical structure, variations in the internal sense of what is male or female, family values, and cultural values
36. exercise behavioral, emotional, economic, and social responsibility for themselves
37. include sexual orientation, gender identity, erotic preferences, and sexual lifestyles
38. chromosomal gender, gonadal gender, internal organs, and external genital appearance
39. ridiculed and humiliated; in constant jeopardy over getting and keeping a job; evicted without cause from restaurants and stores; denied housing; refused medical treatment, even to save a life
40. include several or many partners, nudism, swinging, group sex, fetishism, sexual sadism, and sexual masochism
41. family, culture, religion, and personal expectations and ethics
42. heart disease, diabetes mellitus, joint disease, cancer, and mental disorders
43. (1) Roger has an STI that needs to be treated as soon as possible. (2) The girl's sore throat could be from oral sex and she also needs to be treated for an STI. (3) The clinic will need to treat the teenagers with antibiotics and get a list of their sexual partners so they can all be treated so they do not spread it to other partners. (4) The second girl is also infected and may be pregnant. These teenagers need to have a sexual education course so they understand the dangers of unprotected sex and the consequences of their acts.
44. c. *Rationale:* This is the best answer since human sexuality means different things to different people and evolves as we age and mature.
45. a. *Rationale:* "Normal" sexual expression can vary among cultures and religions, and there are no normal, universal sexual behaviors.
46. b. *Rationale:* Sexuality is developed before birth and continues throughout life.
47. d. *Rationale:* Cramping, lower abdominal pain radiating to the back and upper thighs, nausea, vomiting, diarrhea, and headaches are symptoms of painful menstruation.
48. c. *Rationale:* Adolescents do not practice safe sex and often are with multiple partners, causing an increase in sexually transmitted infections.
49. a. *Rationale:* Individuals can be the best judge of their sexual health and how they feel about it and the changes they go through as they age.
50. b. *Rationale:* In order to form any relationships, you must have a positive self-concept.
51. c. *Rationale:* Sexually healthy people engage in activities that they freely choose for self-pleasuring and shared-pleasuring activities. They have the right and the freedom to make these choices.

52. d. *Rationale:* Sexual orientation is normally male or female, but some individuals are attracted to certain qualities in both males and females.
53. a. *Rationale:* Self-gratification and self-stimulation are ways we discover our erotic feelings and learn about our sexual response.
54. a. *Rationale:* Severe trauma can lead to a phobic response to sexual activity.
55. b. *Rationale:* Sexual activity should bring pleasure to both partners as well as a release for tension.
56. d. *Rationale:* This is the absence of voluntary control of ejaculation.
57. b. *Rationale:* Toxic shock is caused by a form of *Staphylococcus aureus.* If hands are not cleaned before inserting a tampon, this life-threatening problem can result. Also the perineal area must be kept clean and wiped from front to back to prevent *E. coli* from getting into the vaginal area.
58. b. *Rationale:* Medications can have a negative side effect and antidepressants may slow ejaculation.

Chapter 29

1. g   2. o   3. f   4. i   5. k   6. d
7. n   8. m   9. a   10. c   11. e   12. j
13. l   14. b   15. h
16. meaning, value, transcendence, connecting, becoming
17. life experiences, coping skills, social supports, and individual belief systems
18. connectedness with self, others, higher power, all life, nature, and the universe that transcends and empowers the self
19. by conducting an inner dialogue with a higher power or with oneself through prayer or meditation, by analyzing dreams, by communing with nature, or by experiencing the inspiration of art
20. having a medical diagnosis of a terminal or debilitating disease, experiencing pain, experiencing the loss of a body part or function, or experiencing a miscarriage or stillbirth
21. recommendation for blood transfusions, abortion, surgery, dietary restrictions, amputation of a body part, or isolation
22. "a way of living, a lifestyle that views and lives life as purposeful and pleasurable, that seeks out life-sustaining and life-enriching options to be chosen freely at every opportunity, and that sinks its roots deeply into spiritual values and/or specific religious beliefs"
23. joy and laughter, participation in religious services and associated fellowship gatherings and activities, and expression of compassion, empathy, forgiveness, and hope
24. a sense of community bound by common beliefs; the collective study of scripture; the performance of ritual; the use of disciplines and practices, commandments, and sacraments; and ways of taking care of the person's spirit
25. birth, transition from childhood to adulthood, marriage, illness, and death
26. Seek a basic understanding of clients' spiritual needs, resources, and preferences. Follow the client's expressed wishes regarding spiritual care. Do not prescribe or urge clients to adopt certain spiritual beliefs or practices, and do not pressure them to relinquish such beliefs or practices. Strive to understand personal spirituality and how it influences caregiving. Provide spiritual care in a way that is consonant with personal beliefs.
27. fasting, reflection, and prayer
28. jewelry, medals, amulets, icons, totems, or body ornamentation
29. worn to pronounce one's faith, to remind the practitioner of the faith, to provide spiritual protection, or to be a source of comfort or strength
30. ritual, petitionary, colloquial, meditational
31. For what purpose am I sharing my beliefs or practices? By doing so, am I meeting my needs or my client's? Is my spiritual care reflecting a spiritual assessment? Am I preying on a vulnerable client? Am I offering my beliefs or practices in a manner that allows my client comfortably to refuse? Does my spiritual care hurt or contribute to a therapeutic relationship with the client?
32. Helping clients to keep in touch with nature and maintain a sense of wonder is also a form of spiritual care. Examples include recognizing the seasons, the emergence of flowers in spring, the phases of the moon, the migrations of birds, and the unchanging stars.
33. (1) Often when people get sick, they turn to a higher power to help them, even bargaining to get them through the illness. (2) He has three children. Even though he is divorced, he is still young and could start life over with someone else. (3) A clergy may be able to help him focus on himself, give him hope through prayer, and improve his chances for survival through a belief system. (4) Nurses need to consider specific religious practices that will affect nursing care. The nurse's presence is often the best and sometimes the only intervention to support a client who suffers under circumstances that medical interventions cannot address.
34. a. *Rationale:* We all have spiritual needs. Nurses need to be able to understand the different forms of religion and help clients with their spiritual needs without projecting their own beliefs onto the clients.
35. b. *Rationale:* Spirit titer is influenced by numerous factors, such as life experiences, coping skills, social supports, and individual belief systems. If it is not strong, it can cause depression.
36. c. *Rationale:* Often, clients who do not believe in or worship a divine being will question why they are sick or even turn to prayer for an answer. Nurses need to guide them through this time. Clergy for all denominations is usually on call to assist.

37. d. *Rationale:* Religion has many forms but each is organized with set patterns to follow.
38. a. *Rationale:* People follow their heritage and culture norms, and this country was founded on religious freedom by each religious group.
39. a. *Rationale:* In the absence of hope, the client gives up, losing spirit, and illness is likely to progress more rapidly.
40. b. *Rationale:* When a nurse uses the same terms as the client, the client will be able to relate and form a relationship that can be therapeutic.
41. d. *Rationale:* Muslims pray at least five times a day, and nurses need to provide privacy and time to allow clients the freedom to practice their spirituality.
42. c. *Rationale:* All religions except these two view the Sabbath as Sunday.
43. c. *Rationale:* Blood transfusions are in conflict with the religious admonitions of Jehovah's Witnesses.
44. a. *Rationale:* This assessment is taken at the end of the regular assessment and only general questions can be asked.
45. b. *Rationale:* Prayer can be done anywhere and privately. It provides the connection with a higher power.
46. c. *Rationale:* Although care is necessary it can be arranged around spiritual needs. The nurse needs to provide the opportunity and privacy for clients to pray.
47. b. *Rationale:* The nurse and religious counselor can work together to meet the client's needs.

Chapter 30

1. h   2. f   3. k   4. n   5. o   6. q
7. w   8. r   9. v   10. i   11. p   12. c
13. e   14. t   15. s   16. g   17. u   18. l
19. b   20. y   21. m   22. x   23. a   24. j
25. d

26. coping strategies, coping responses, or coping mechanisms
27. internal, external, developmental, and situational
28. physical, emotional, intellectual, social, and spiritual
29. stimulus based, response based, and transaction based
30. gastrointestinal tract, the adrenal glands, and the lymphatic structures
31. physiologic, psychologic, or cognitive
32. anxiety, fear, anger, depression, and unconscious ego defense mechanisms
33. Mild anxiety produces a slight arousal state that enhances perception, learning, and productive abilities. Most healthy people experience mild anxiety, perhaps as a feeling of mild restlessness that prompts a person to seek information and ask questions. Moderate anxiety increases the arousal state to a point where the person expresses feelings of tension, nervousness, or concern. Perceptual abilities are narrowed. Attention is focused more on a particular aspect of a situation than on peripheral activities. Severe anxiety consumes most of the person's energies and requires intervention. Perception is further decreased. The person, unable to focus on what is really happening, focuses on only one specific detail of the situation generating the anxiety. Panic is an overpowering, frightening level of anxiety causing the person to lose control. It is less frequently experienced than other levels of anxiety. The perception of a panicked person can be affected to the degree that the person distorts events.
34. The source of anxiety may not be identifiable; the source of fear is identifiable. Anxiety is related to the future, that is, to an anticipated event. Fear is related to the present. Anxiety is vague, whereas fear is definite. Anxiety is the result of psychologic or emotional conflict; fear is the result of a discrete physical or psychologic entity.
35. sadness, despair, dejection, lack of worth, or emptiness
36. tiredness, sadness, emptiness, or numbness
37. irritability, inability to concentrate, difficulty making decisions, loss of sexual desire, crying, sleep disturbance, and social withdrawal
38. include loss of appetite, weight loss, constipation, headache, and dizziness
39. problem-focused and emotion-focused coping
40. using alcoholic beverages or drugs, daydreaming and fantasizing, relying on the belief that everything will work out, and giving in to others to avoid anger
41. alter the stressor, adapt to the stressor, or avoid the stressor
42. the number, duration, and intensity of the stressors; past experiences of the individual; support systems available to the individual; personal qualities of the person
43. nursing history, and physical examination of the client for indicators of stress or stress-related health problems
44. anxiety, depression, weight loss, difficulties in swallowing, vomiting, fatigue, headaches, dizziness, fainting, blurred vision, skin rashes, excessive sweating, menstrual disturbances, palpitations, chest pain, and dyspnea
45. (1) Helen is suffering from major depression. (2) The type of depression is known as situational depression that was brought on by her husband's illness and death. (3) The doctor could have offered her help through therapy and talking with someone who would understand what she was going through. All too often doctors prescribe medications to clients and they often do not produce the desired effect. (4) Nurses can listen and provide an outlet. It is often easier to talk to strangers, especially when you will probably not see that person again.
46. b. *Rationale:* Internal stressors cause disease and illnesses.
47. d. *Rationale:* We cannot control events that will happen throughout our lives or whether they are happy or sad, so with each situation our bodies go through stress. The degree to which these events have positive

or negative effects can depend on an individual's developmental stage and coping strategies.

48. a. *Rationale:* In stimulus-based stress models, stress is defined as a stimulus, a life event, or a set of circumstances that arouses physiologic and/or psychologic reactions. These reactions can cause illness.
49. c. *Rationale:* Scales have been developed to rate the degree of stress an event can cause, but each person is different and will be affected differently. Stress is highly individual.
50. c. *Rationale:* Because stress is a state of the body, it can be observed only by the changes it produces in the body. The release of hormones can change both the structure and chemical composition.
51. a. *Rationale:* Responses to stress vary depending on the individual's perception of events, which can then affect the systems of the body.
52. b. *Rationale:* Anxiety is a state of mental uneasiness, apprehension, dread, or foreboding or a feeling of helplessness related to an impending or anticipated unidentified threat to self or significant relationships.
53. c. *Rationale:* It is an emotional state consisting of a subjective feeling of animosity or strong displeasure.
54. d. *Rationale*: If the anger persists unabated, violence and destructiveness will result.
55. b. *Rationale:* Getting anger out into the open prevents an emotional buildup and can prevent violence.
56. a. *Rationale:* Clients with prolonged depression are unable to bring themselves out of it without help and that usually requires the use of medications.
57. b. *Rationale:* Defense mechanisms are coping mechanisms that will ultimately solve the problem.
58. d. *Rationale:* Assess the situation or problem, analyze or define it, choose an alternative, carry out the selected alternative, and evaluate whether the solution is successful.
59. a. *Rationale:* Nurses need to understand how anger affects them so they can work with the clients' anger issues.
60. c. *Rationale:* When a nurse feels physically threatened, getting away from the situation may be the only answer if no one is around to assist.
61. b. *Rationale:* Nurses need to be prepared to provide sensitive, skilled, and supportive care to all clients no matter what the loss.
62. c. *Rationale:* Confrontation is the most upsetting stage, although each stage is difficult.
63. c. *Rationale:* Hindus prefer cremation and cast the ashes in a holy river. Cremation is becoming more common, especially in the Christian religions.
64. d. *Rationale:* Hearing is the last sense that is lost.

Chapter 31

1. h   2. o   3. g   4. k   5. q   6. l
7. b   8. m   9. s   10. r   11. t   12. v
13. w   14. a   15. y   16. f   17. z   18. i
19. u   20. d   21. x   22. p   23. n   24. j
25. e   26. c
27. weight and exercise
28. body alignment (posture), joint mobility, balance, and coordinated movement
29. mood, self-esteem, and personality
30. lung expansion and promotes efficient circulatory, renal, and gastrointestinal functions
31. genetic makeup, developmental patterns, the presence or absence of disease, and physical activity
32. muscle tone, mass, and strength, and maintain joint flexibility and circulation
33. abdominal, gluteal, and quadriceps muscles; also to maintain strength in immobilized muscles in casts or traction; and for endurance training
34. increases joint flexibility, stability, and range of motion and improves blood supply to the joint
35. eliminate toxins with deeper breathing, enhance problem solving and emotional stability
36. muscle tone and bone density decrease, joints lose flexibility, reaction time slows, and bone mass decreases
37. values, geographic location, and cultural role expectations
38. degree of fun or challenge of any given activity; use of music; opportunities for socializing and group cohesion and having an exercise partner; positive sensations of the exercise experience; pleasurable feelings associated with increased stress reduction; increased energy and fitness; mastering the activity; goal setting and progress; daily logs or weekly written schedules; competition with oneself or others; promotion of a sense of accomplishment; weight management; emphasis on self-talk about how exercise will prevent fatigue, depression, weight gain, or anxiety; and the need to explore less intense and challenging, non-competitive activities
39. nervous system, musculoskeletal system, cardiovascular system, respiratory system, and vestibular apparatus
40. assessment methods of inspection, palpation, and auscultation; checks results of laboratory tests; and takes measurements, including body weight, fluid intake, and fluid output
41. stop smoking, regular movement, stretching, drink fluids, and keep legs uncrossed
42. increased tolerance for physical activity, restored or improved capability to ambulate and/or participate in ADLs, absence of injury from falling or improper use of body mechanics, enhanced physical fitness, absence of any complications associated with immobility, and improved social, emotional, and intellectual well-being
43. low back pain, herniated discs, strained muscles, pulled and/or torn ligaments, and disc degradation

44. thighs, knees, upper and lower arms, abdomen, and pelvis
45. sagging mattress, a mattress that is too soft, or an underfilled waterbed
46. pallor, diaphoresis, nausea, tachycardia, and dizziness
47. to cope with daily stresses, to prevent fatigue, to conserve energy, to restore the mind and body, to enjoy life more fully, and to enhance daytime functioning
48. apathy, depression, irritability, confusion, disorientation, hallucinations, impaired memory, and paranoia
49. (1) She will need to be turned and positioned and pillows placed to make her comfortable. She should be able to assist with an over-the-bed patient helper. (2) When the nurse is helping her to position, she should have help and possibly use mechanical assistance and always use good body mechanics. (3) Pillows can be used to support other painful joints and keep the pressure off with positioning. (4) Sleep is needed for her body to heal. Recuperative sleep will also give her energy to get through the therapy she needs to regain the use of her knee.
50. c. *Rationale:* Exercise and activity are an essential component of health, and aging adults need to remain active to maintain health.
51. a. *Rationale:* With 24 years of data collection, mortality rates have been lowest for women who are lean *and* active. Exercise and nutrition are keys to good health and longevity.
52. c. *Rationale:* The ability to move freely, easily, rhythmically, and purposefully in the environment is essential for quality of life.
53. d. *Rationale:* It operates movement, not muscles.
54. d. *Rationale:* Although all these answers promote strong bones, weight-bearing exercises help maintain strength and density.
55. c. *Rationale:* Bones and muscles need to be used and exercised to maintain strength and agility.
56. c. *Rationale:* Bed rest may delay recovery or actually harm clients.
57. b. *Rationale:* Nurses need to evaluate clients for risks of immobility and to prevent it.
58. a. *Rationale:* Body mechanics (ergonomics) helps to reduce musculoskeletal injuries during lifting, transferring, and repositioning.
59. b. *Rationale:* The base of support is enlarged in the direction in which the movement is to be produced or opposed.
60. d. *Rationale:* Clients with problems breathing need to be in the best position to expand the lungs, and the Fowler position is the best one to accomplish that. In this position, gravity pulls the diaphragm downward, allowing greater chest expansion and lung ventilation.
61. b. *Rationale:* Clients with cardiac or respiratory problems find the prone position confining and suffocating because chest expansion is inhibited during respirations.
62. d. *Rationale:* Flexion reduces lordosis and promotes good back alignment.
63. a. *Rationale:* Sims' is the only correct answer.
64. c. *Rationale:* An intact cerebral cortex and reticular formation are necessary for the regulation of sleep and waking states.
65. d. *Rationale:* A person preoccupied with personal problems may be unable to relax sufficiently to get to sleep.
66. a. *Rationale:* If a sleep pattern is established it will eventually become a habit to go to bed and get up at the same time every day.

Chapter 32

1. d   2. w   3. i   4. j   5. k   6. m
7. q   8. a   9. p   10. v   11. b   12. y
13. u   14. g   15. r   16. t   17. e   18. c
19. x   20. n   21. l   22. f   23. h   24. o
25. z   26. s
27. water, carbohydrates, proteins, fats, vitamins, and minerals
28. providing energy for body processes and movement, providing structural material for body tissues, and regulating body processes
29. carbon (C), hydrogen (H), and oxygen (O)
30. simple carbohydrates (sugars) and complex carbohydrates (starches and fiber)
31. glucose, fructose, and galactose
32. carbon, hydrogen, oxygen, and nitrogen
33. histidine, isoleucine, leucine, lysine, methionine, phenylalanine, tryptophan, threonine, and valine
34. alanine, aspartic acid, cystine, glutamic acid, glycine, hydroxyproline, proline, serine, and tyrosine
35. complete proteins, partially complete proteins, or incomplete proteins
36. proteolytic enzymes trypsin, chymotrypsin, and carboxypeptidase
37. building tissue, breaking down tissue, and nitrogen balance
38. vitamins C and B–complex
39. vitamins A, D, E, and K
40. developmental considerations, gender, ethnicity and culture, beliefs about food, personal preferences, religious practices, lifestyle, economics, medications and therapies, health, alcohol consumption, advertising, and psychologic factors
41. Make mealtime a pleasant time by avoiding tensions at the table and discussions of bad behavior. Offer a variety of simple, attractive foods in small portions, and avoid meals that combine foods into one dish, such as a stew. Do not use food as a reward or punish a child who does not eat. Schedule meals, sleep, and snack times that will allow for optimum appetite and behavior. Avoid the routine use of sweet desserts.

42. lack of transportation, poor access to stores, inability to prepare the food, do not want to cook for themselves, or eat alone
43. Consume nutrient-dense foods within caloric needs. Maintain weight in a healthy range. Engage in regular physical activity. Consume recommended amounts of fruit, vegetables, whole grains, and milk each day. Keep total fat intake within 20% to 35% of total calories and less than 10% from saturated fatty acids. Consume less than 2,300 mg of sodium per day and add potassium-rich foods. Drink alcohol in moderation.
44. activity, moderation, personalization, proportionality, variety, and gradual improvement
45. economic, health, religious, ethical, or ecologic reasons
46. marked weight loss, generalized weakness, altered functional abilities, delayed wound healing, increased susceptibility to infection, decreased immunocompetence, impaired pulmonary function, and prolonged length of hospitalization
47. (1) He will need to have more calories added to his diet to heal but not too many that will cause him to gain weight. (2) As an Orthodox Jew, he will need to have only kosher foods and no pork in his diet. (3) He will need to have vitamins and minerals, especially iron because of his blood loss and vitamin C to aid in healing. He will also need to have fiber in his diet and plenty of fluids so he does not become constipated. (4) Families can bring in food, but the calories will need to be calculated by looking at the foods that they bring in. It will be important to have enough protein in his diet.
48. c. *Rationale:* Water makes up 60% of the body and needs to be replaced frequently.
49. d. *Rationale:* Fiber is roughage that is not digested but helps to carry processed foods and waste products through the gastrointestinal system.
50. b. *Rationale:* Processed carbohydrate foods are relatively low in nutrients and high in calories.
51. a. *Rationale:* Excess glucose that cannot be used as energy or converted for storage is converted to fat.
52. c. *Rationale:* The body requires amino acids whether they come from meat or plant proteins. A balanced ratio of amino acids can be achieved if an appropriate mixture of plant proteins is provided in the diet.
53. d. *Rationale:* Pepsin is an enzyme in the mouth that breaks down protein.
54. b. *Rationale:* They are absorbed by active transport through the small intestine and into the portal blood circulation.
55. c. *Rationale:* The body does not store amino acids, but they need to be replaced daily.
56. d. *Rationale:* Nitrogen balance reflects the status of protein nutrition in the body.
57. c. *Rationale:* Lipids can be fats or oils, and they contain a higher proportion of hydrogen.
58. b. *Rationale:* Glycerides are the simplest and most common forms.
59. c. *Rationale:* Bile acids are created from cholesterol.
60. a. *Rationale:* Only glycerol can be converted to glucose, the only substance that feeds the body's cells.
61. a. *Rationale:* Water-soluble vitamins cannot be stored in the body. They are carried out in the urine.
62. d. *Rationale:* Fat-soluble vitamins are stored in the fat and can become toxic, but vitamins E and K need to be replaced more often.
63. d. *Rationale:* Foods eaten create energy to maintain activities.
64. a. *Rationale:* Hypertension is a major concern that can be resolved by losing weight. Even as little as 5 pounds can make a difference.
65. b. *Rationale:* Excess body weight increases the stress on body organs and predisposes people to chronic health problems.
66. d. *Rationale:* Triceps are the most common site.
67. b. *Rationale:* Albumin is one of the most common visceral proteins and is checked to see how much protein has been ingested.

Chapter 33

1. g 2. j 3. l 4. r 5. p 6. m
7. t 8. b 9. n 10. u 11. q 12. o
13. v 14. s 15. e 16. x 17. a 18. h
19. w 20. d 21. z 22. i 23. f 24. y
25. k 26. c

27. social culture, personal habits, and physical abilities
28. social propriety of leaving to urinate, the availability of a private clean facility, and initial bladder training
29. functioning of the kidneys, ureters, urinary bladder, urethra, and pelvic floor
30. water, electrolytes, glucose, amino acids, and metabolic wastes
31. an inner mucous layer; a connective tissue layer; three layers of smooth muscle fibers, some of which extend lengthwise, some obliquely, and some more or less circularly; and an outer serous layer
32. compromise the kidney's ability to filter, maintain acid–base balance, and maintain electrolyte balance
33. urinary urgency and urinary frequency
34. privacy, normal position, sufficient time, and, occasionally, running water
35. diabetes mellitus, diabetes insipidus, and chronic nephritis
36. cause excessive fluid loss, leading to intense thirst, dehydration, and weight loss
37. hemodialysis and peritoneal dialysis
38. frequency, nocturia, urgency, and dysuria
39. enuresis, incontinence, retention, and neurogenic bladder

40. urinary tract infections, urethritis, pregnancy, hypercalcemia, volume overload, delirium, restricted mobility, stool impaction, and psychologic causes
41. polyuria, exposure to irritants, infection, urinary retention, use of pharmaceuticals, stool impaction or constipation, atrophic urethritis or vaginitis, restricted mobility or dexterity, psychologic conditions, and delirium or acute confused state
42. stress, urge, reflex, retention with overflow, and functional incontinence
43. sodium, chloride, potassium, sulfate, magnesium, and phosphorus
44. collecting urine specimens, measuring specific gravity, and visualization procedures
45. Maintain or restore a normal voiding pattern. Regain normal urine output. Prevent associated risks such as infection, skin breakdown, fluid and electrolyte imbalance, and lowered self-esteem. Perform toilet activities independently with or without assistive devices. Contain urine with the appropriate device, catheter, ostomy appliance, or absorbent product.
46. (1) No matter what the age, any changes in the body and its functions will cause a disturbance in body image. Since she will not be providing care for herself, she may not be able to look at or to touch the stoma and appliance. (2) This would depend on the facility's policy. (3) There may be a risk of infection because the stomas provide direct access for microorganisms. (4) The wound ostomy continence nurse (WOCN) is the best person to identify strategies for management of stoma and peristomal problems and to provide care, but other nurses can also be trained to provide necessary care unless a problem arises.
47. b. *Rationale:* The kidneys have millions of nephrons that filter the blood and remove metabolic wastes.
48. a. *Rationale:* The body reabsorbs products that are necessary to maintain fluid and electrolyte balance.
49. d. *Rationale:* The urinary bladder stores and excretes urine.
50. b. *Rationale:* Nocturnal enuresis occurs because the client fails to awaken when the bladder empties.
51. c. *Rationale:* Problems with the kidneys slowing the excretion of drugs can cause them to accumulate, causing a toxic effect.
52. a. *Rationale:* The capacity of the bladder and its ability to completely empty diminish with age, and the urine that sits in the bladder can cause an infection.
53. b. *Rationale:* Holding urine in the bladder can cause bladder infections. If urine is allowed to back up into the ureters, it can cause a kidney infection.
54. d. *Rationale:* Alcoholic beverages, especially beer, increase fluid output and can actually dehydrate the body.
55. d. *Rationale:* Foods and medications can turn urine a different color than normal or change the odor of urine.
56. c. *Rationale:* Diuretics increase urinary output.
57. c. *Rationale:* The detrusor muscle is needed so the bladder can fill adequately and empty completely, but the contributor is the pelvic muscle.
58. c. *Rationale:* Urea and creatinine are eliminated by the kidneys through filtration and tubular secretion.
59. a. *Rationale:* Infections from indwelling catheters are common, and strict sterile conditions must be observed as well as keeping the area around the meatus clean.
60. c. *Rationale:* The ureters remain connected to the bladder, and the bladder wall is surgically attached to an opening in the skin below the navel forming an incontinent stoma.
61. c. *Rationale:* Urine irritates the skin and a well-fitting appliance is vital.
62. b. *Rationale:* Clients who have surgical alterations to urinary systems will need to accept the changes and the altered body image.

Chapter 34

1. d   2. i   3. k   4. n   5. l   6. p
7. r   8. u   9. w   10. a   11. s   12. f
13. g   14. q   15. b   16. j   17. v   18. t
19. o   20. e   21. m   22. x   23. h   24. c

25. cecum; ascending, transverse, and descending colons; sigmoid colon; rectum; and anus
26. absorption of water and nutrients, the mucoid protection of the intestinal wall, and fecal elimination
27. carbon dioxide, methane, hydrogen, oxygen, and nitrogen
28. fluid intake and output, activity, psychologic factors, lifestyle, medications and medical procedures, and disease
29. adequate roughage in the diet, adequate exercise, and six to eight glasses of fluid daily
30. cabbage, onions, cauliflower, bananas, apples, bran, prunes, figs, chocolate, alcohol, cheese, pasta, eggs, and lean meat
31. lack of exercise, immobility, or impaired neurologic functioning
32. constipation, diarrhea, bowel incontinence, and flatulence
33. insufficient fiber intake, insufficient fluid intake, insufficient activity or immobility, irregular defecation habits, change in daily routine, lack of privacy, chronic use of laxatives or enemas, irritable bowel syndrome, pelvic floor dysfunction or muscle damage, poor motility or slow transit, neurologic conditions, emotional disturbances such as depression or mental confusion, and medications such as opioids, iron supplements, antihistamines, antacids, and antidepressants
34. heart disease, brain injuries, or respiratory disease

35.

Psychologic stress	Increased intestinal motility and mucus secretion
Medications	Inflammation and infection of mucosa due to overgrowth of pathogenic intestinal microorganisms
Antibiotics	Irritation of intestinal mucosa
Iron	Irritation of intestinal mucosa
Cathartics	Incomplete digestion of food or fluid
Allergy to food, fluid, drugs	Increased intestinal motility and mucus secretion
Intolerance of food or fluid	Reduced absorption of fluids
Diseases of the colon	Inflammation of the mucosa often leading to ulcer formation

36. partial and major
37. action of bacteria on the chyme in the large intestine, swallowed air, and gas that diffuses between the bloodstream and the intestine
38. their status as permanent or temporary, their anatomic location, and the construction of the stoma, the opening created in the abdominal wall by the ostomy
39. single, loop, divided, or double-barreled
40. color, consistency, shape, amount, odor, and the presence of abnormal constituents
41. Maintain or restore normal bowel elimination pattern. Maintain or regain normal stool consistency. Prevent associated risks such as fluid and electrolyte imbalance, skin breakdown, abdominal distention, and pain.
42. the provision of privacy, timing, nutrition and fluids, exercise, and positioning
43. cathartics and laxatives, antidiarrheals, and antiflatulents
44. nausea, cramps, colic, vomiting, or undiagnosed abdominal pain
45. (1) She will need to know how to keep the stoma clean and replace the appliance as needed and empty the pouch. She will also need to be taught how to minimize the odor and also how to dress so the appliance is comfortable. (2) She was probably better off having the surgery. If she had continued to have fecal drainage in the vaginal area, the tissue would have eroded away. This would have made the fistula larger, and it could have extended into other areas. (3) The tissue was friable because the fecal drainage is very caustic with digestive enzymes and breaks down healthy tissue. (4) Sandy could benefit from having others with colostomies to talk to and to share ideas about surviving with a colostomy.
46. a. *Rationale:* It is located at the junction of the ileum of the small intestine and the first part of the large intestine and controls the chyme.
47. c. *Rationale:* A squeeze-like action called peristaltic waves moves food waste products through the intestines.
48. b. *Rationale:* When the body is stopped from defecating the colon will reabsorb more of the fluid, making the stool harder and drier.
49. a. *Rationale:* Fecal matter is brown because of the presence of stercobilin and urobilin and also the E. coli bacteria.
50. c. *Rationale:* Older adults often miss the important keys to maintain bowel functioning. They may drink less water and walk less. They often do not eat fiber-containing foods, and they may have weak muscles.
51. c. *Rationale:* After meals, especially breakfast, the reflex is the strongest.
52. c. *Rationale:* Overuse of laxatives can create a dependency on them and can also inhibit the functioning of the muscles if waste is forced through in a liquid state.
53. d. *Rationale:* A mass or collection of hardened feces in the folds of the rectum stops normal defecation but allows liquid stool to bypass the impaction.
54. b. *Rationale:* Rapid passage of chyme reduces the time available for the large intestine to reabsorb water and electrolytes, forcing the body to have fatigue, weakness, malaise, and emaciation from prolonged diarrhea.
55. d. *Rationale:* Diarrhea can be caused from irritants in the intestinal tract. Flushing out those irritants can be protective to the body if it is not prolonged.
56. a. *Rationale:* The position at the bowel would determine whether stool is liquid or formed.
57. b. *Rationale:* Stools from a sigmoidostomy are of normal or formed consistency, and the frequency of discharge can be regulated.
58. a. *Rationale:* A loop stoma has two openings: the proximal or afferent end, which is active, and the distal or efferent end, which is inactive.
59. b. *Rationale:* Constant use of laxatives weakens the muscles and the urge to defecate and can also remove nutrition that should be absorbed by the body.
60. a. *Rationale:* Before the water moves from the colon, it stimulates peristalsis and defecation.

© 2011 by Pearson Education, Inc.

61. c. *Rationale:* During digital disimpaction the bowel mucosa can be injured, and it can cause vagal stimulation that can cause an arrhythmia.

Chapter 35

1. g   2. i   3. k   4. m   5. o   6. c
7. p   8. u   9. v   10. z   11. e   12. a
13. s   14. t   15. r   16. w   17. y   18. x
19. q   20. j   21. b   22. n   23. f   24. l
25. h   26. d

27. pulmonary ventilation or breathing; the movement of air between the atmosphere and the alveoli of the lungs as we inhale and exhale; gas exchange, which involves diffusion of oxygen and carbon dioxide between the alveoli and pulmonary capillaries; and transport of oxygen from the lungs to the tissues, and carbon dioxide from the tissues to the lungs
28. clear airways, an intact central nervous system and respiratory center, an intact thoracic cavity capable of expanding and contracting, adequate pulmonary compliance and recoil
29. cardiac output, number of erythrocytes, blood hematocrit, and exercise
30. hydrogen, oxygen, and carbon dioxide
31. the anterior neck muscles, intercostal muscles, and muscles of the abdomen
32. age, environment, lifestyle, health status, medications, and stress
33. infection, physical or emotional stress, surgery, anesthesia, or other procedures
34. altitude, heat, cold, and air pollution
35. stinging of the eyes, headache, dizziness, coughing, and choking
36. narcotics, benzodiazepine sedative-hypnotics, and antianxiety drugs
37. dilates the bronchioles, increases blood flow and oxygen delivery to active muscles
38. hypoxia, altered breathing patterns, and obstructed or partially obstructed airway
39. ventilation, diffusion of gases, or transport of gases by the blood
40. eupnea, tachypnea, bradypnea, apnea
41. rate, volume, rhythm, and relative ease or effort of respiration
42. include data about current and past respiratory problems; lifestyle; presence of cough, sputum, or pain; medications for breathing; and presence of risk factors for impaired oxygenation status
43. inspection, palpation, percussion, and auscultation
44. sputum specimens, throat cultures, visualization procedures, venous and arterial blood specimens, and pulmonary function tests
45. Maintain a patent airway. Improve comfort and ease of breathing. Maintain or improve pulmonary ventilation and oxygenation. Improve ability to participate in physical activities. Prevent risks associated with oxygenation problems such as skin and tissue breakdown, syncope, acid–base imbalances, and feelings of hopelessness and social isolation.
46. ensuring a patent airway, positioning, encouraging deep breathing and coughing, ensuring adequate hydration, suctioning, lung inflation techniques, administration of analgesics before deep breathing and coughing, postural drainage, and percussion and vibration
47. positioning the client to allow for maximum chest expansion, encouraging or providing frequent changes in position, encouraging ambulation, and implementing measures that promote comfort
48. dizziness, lightheadedness, drowsiness, nervousness, nausea, vomiting, and stomach pain
49. (1) The smoking and the environment he works in have caused lung damage and compromised his respiratory status. (2) Joe needs to quit smoking and may consider changing careers. His COPD will only get worse unless he makes some lifestyle changes. (3) Oxygen levels should be 100%, but with his compromised lungs he would do well at 90%. However, the oxygen could create more problems and he will only be able to tolerate 1 L via nasal cannula. (4) If he has no other problems with today's DRGs, he will probably be sent home after treatment and lab work with medication and a follow-up with a specialist.
50. a. *Rationale:* The fine hair-like cilia help keep foreign bodies from entering the lungs.
51. b. *Rationale:* Diffusion is the only correct answer.
52. c. *Rationale:* The body's "respiratory center" is actually a number of groups of neurons located in the medulla oblongata and pons of the brain.
53. d. *Rationale:* Surfactant is produced by specialized alveolar cells. It acts like a detergent, reducing the surface tension of alveolar fluid.
54. a. *Rationale:* As the body's activity increases, the need for more oxygen increases the rate of respirations.
55. c. *Rationale:* Slow respiratory rate is called bradypnea.
56. c. *Rationale:* During hyperventilation, the rate and depth of respirations increase, and more CO_2 is eliminated than is produced.
57. a. *Rationale:* Dyspnea is a subjective feeling. The client can report it, but it is not measurable.
58. c. *Rationale:* The chest adapts to chronic respiratory conditions.
59. b. *Rationale:* Although other additives can create side effects, pseudoephedrine causes these problems.
60. a. *Rationale:* Gravity pulls the secretions out with postural drainage treatments.
61. d. *Rationale:* Oxygen is odorless and colorless and can explode when subjected to a spark or flame.
62. c. *Rationale*: A tracheostomy is placed in the neck, so the only method that will be beneficial is a mist collar.

63. a. *Rationale:* This is used exclusively for clients with a pneumothorax who usually have small amounts of fluid.
64. c. *Rationale*: The heart serves as the system pump, moving blood through the vessels to the tissues.
65. a. *Rationale:* Coronary arteries originate at the base of the aorta, branching out to encircle and penetrate the myocardium to feed the muscles of the heart. The blood that flows in and out of the heart does not contribute to keeping the heart alive.
66. d. *Rationale:* A network of specialized cells and pathways known as the cardiac conduction system normally controls the electrical activity and contraction of the heart.
67. c. *Rationale:* Blood carries all the needed nutrients and the oxygen to keep the cells healthy.
68. b. *Rationale:* During middle adulthood, the incidence of hypertension, or an elevated blood pressure, increases significantly.
69. b. *Rationale:* Clients with elevated homocysteine levels may have an increased risk of myocardial infarction, coronary artery disease, cerebrovascular accidents (stroke), and peripheral vascular disease.

Chapter 36

1. y   2. f   3. j   4. l   5. h   6. a
7. c   8. n   9. p   10. t   11. r   12. b
13. v   14. i   15. w   16. u   17. e   18. z
19. s   20. m   21. g   22. q   23. o   24. k
25. x   26. d
27. medium for metabolic reactions within cells; transport nutrients, waste products, and other substances; function as a lubricant, insulator, and shock absorber; and regulate and maintain body temperature
28. intracellular and extracellular
29. oxygen, electrolytes, and glucose
30. oxygen from the lungs, dissolved nutrients from the gastrointestinal tract, excretory products of metabolism
31. age, sex, and body fat
32. cerebrospinal, pericardial, pancreatic, pleural, intraocular, biliary, peritoneal, and synovial fluids
33. sodium, chloride, and bicarbonate
34. vomiting, diarrhea, or gastric suction
35. osmosis, diffusion, filtration, and active transport
36. electrolytes, oxygen, carbon dioxide, glucose, urea, amino acids, and proteins
37. potassium, glucose, and urea
38. urine, insensible loss, noticeable loss through the skin, loss through the intestines in feces
39. illness, trauma, surgery, and medication
40. vomiting, diarrhea, or nasogastric suction
41. kidneys, the endocrine system, the cardiovascular system, the lungs, and the gastrointestinal system
42. blood volume, temperature, pain, stress, and drugs such as opiates and barbiturates
43. maintaining fluid balance, contributing to acid–base regulation, facilitating enzyme reactions, transmitting neuromuscular reactions
44. regulating muscle contraction and relaxation, neuromuscular function, and cardiac function
45. cereal grains, nuts, dried fruit, legumes, green leafy vegetables, dairy products, meat, and fish
46. shortness of breath, chest pain, cough, hypotension, tachycardia, and anxiety after the insertion procedure
47. (1) She has a serious case of gastritis, possibly caused by undercooked fish or *E. coli* from a restaurant employee who failed to wash their hands following defecation. (2) She will need to have fluids and electrolytes replaced. (3) She may have a dysrythmia due to the loss of electrolytes from vomiting and diarrhea. (4) Many tests can be ordered but the most important would be blood work to see what she is low in. Then if the problem does not clear up, other tests might include barium enemas, upper GIs, and checking the stool for ova and parasites. If this was food poisoning, it should be reported to the health department and they could check the restaurant for problems.
48. c. *Rationale:* Infants have more water incorporated in their weight than any other age group.
49. b. *Rationale:* Extracellular is the only correct answer.
50. a. *Rationale:* Plasma is the part of blood without the erythrocytes.
51. d. *Rationale:* This is the only correct answer.
52. b. *Rationale:* Osmosis occurs when the concentration of solutes on one side of a selectively permeable membrane is higher than on the other side.
53. a. *Rationale:* The lungs can work very quickly and the kidneys work much more slowly to regulate balance.
54. c. *Rationale:* This causes the collecting ducts to become more permeable to water.
55. c. *Rationale:* Potassium is involved in maintaining acid–base balance and it contributes to intracellular enzyme reactions.
56. c. *Rationale:* Although cheese may have calcium, not all cheeses are made with milk. The best answer is milk.
57. c. *Rationale:* This is one of the six measurements commonly used in interpreting arterial blood gases.
58. c. *Rationale:* This solution has the same concentration of solutes as blood plasma.
59. b. *Rationale:* A PICC line eliminates the risk of pneumothorax and is safer to use for the client in a home setting.
60. a. *Rationale:* These age groups are the most susceptible to excess fluids.
61. d. *Rationale:* This is the only fluid that will not damage the blood components. Others may cause the blood cells to clump or cause clotting.
62. c. *Rationale:* The thirst mechanism is located in the brain. Osmotic pressure stimulates the thirst center so the person will drink to replace the necessary fluid.

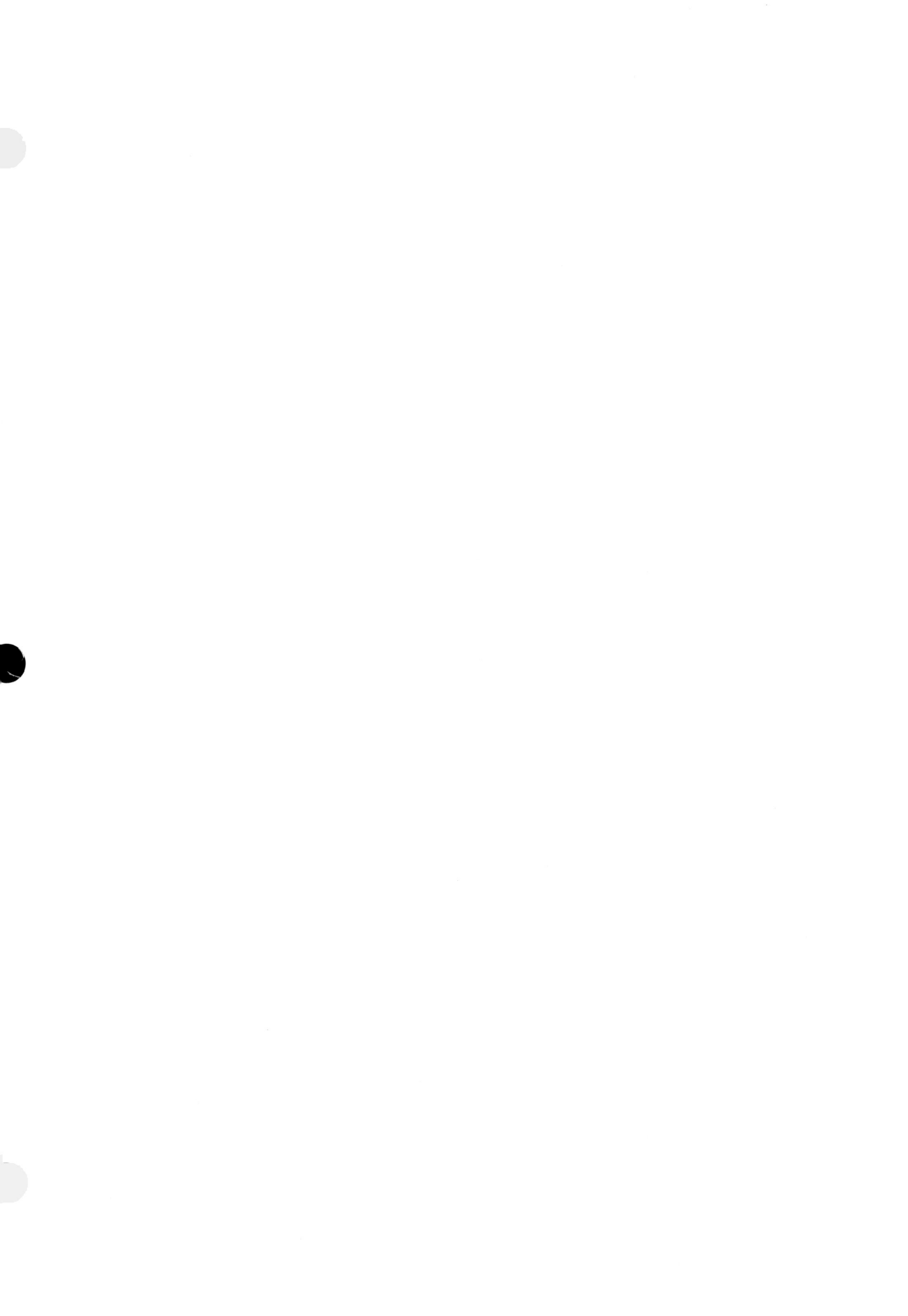

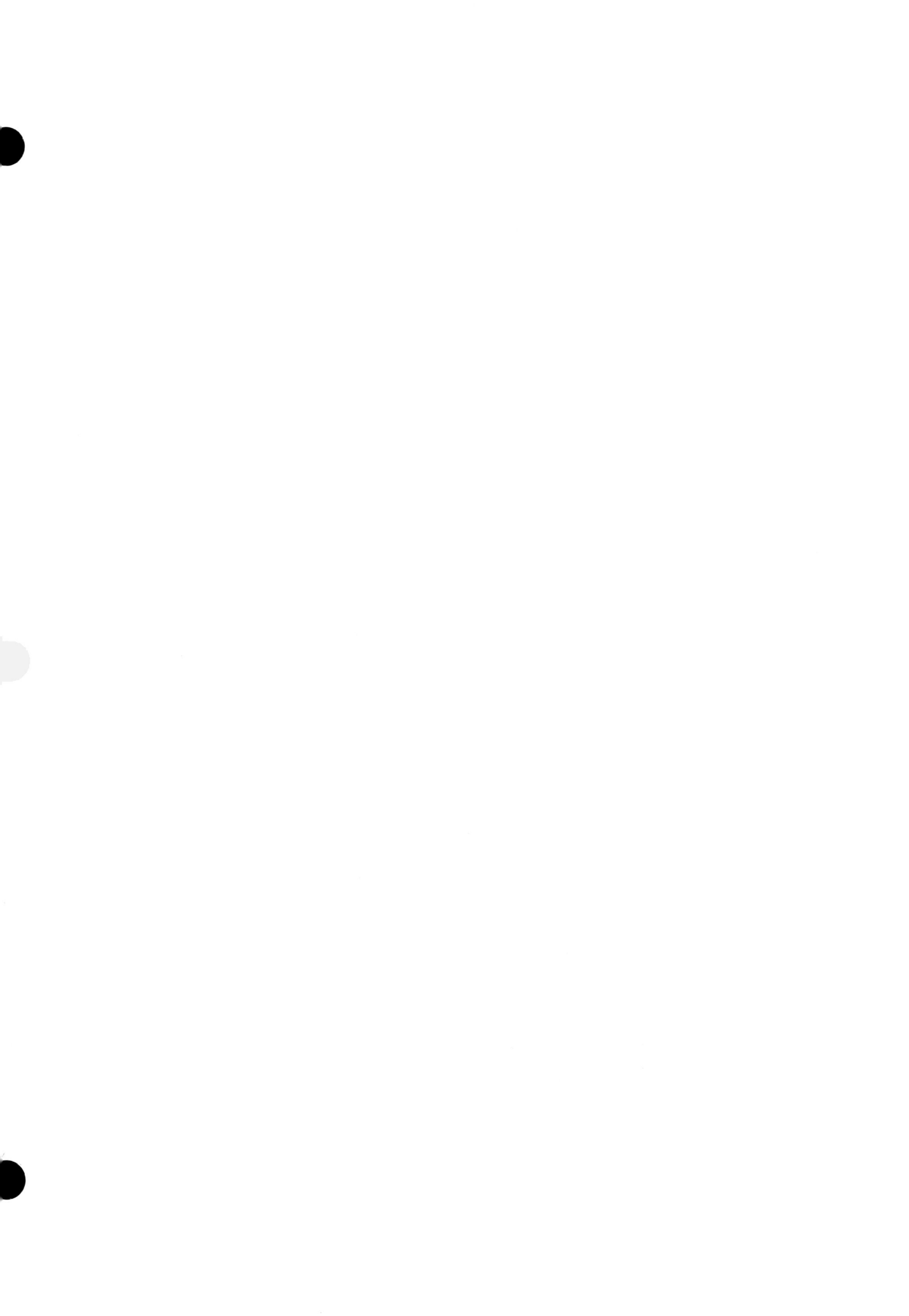

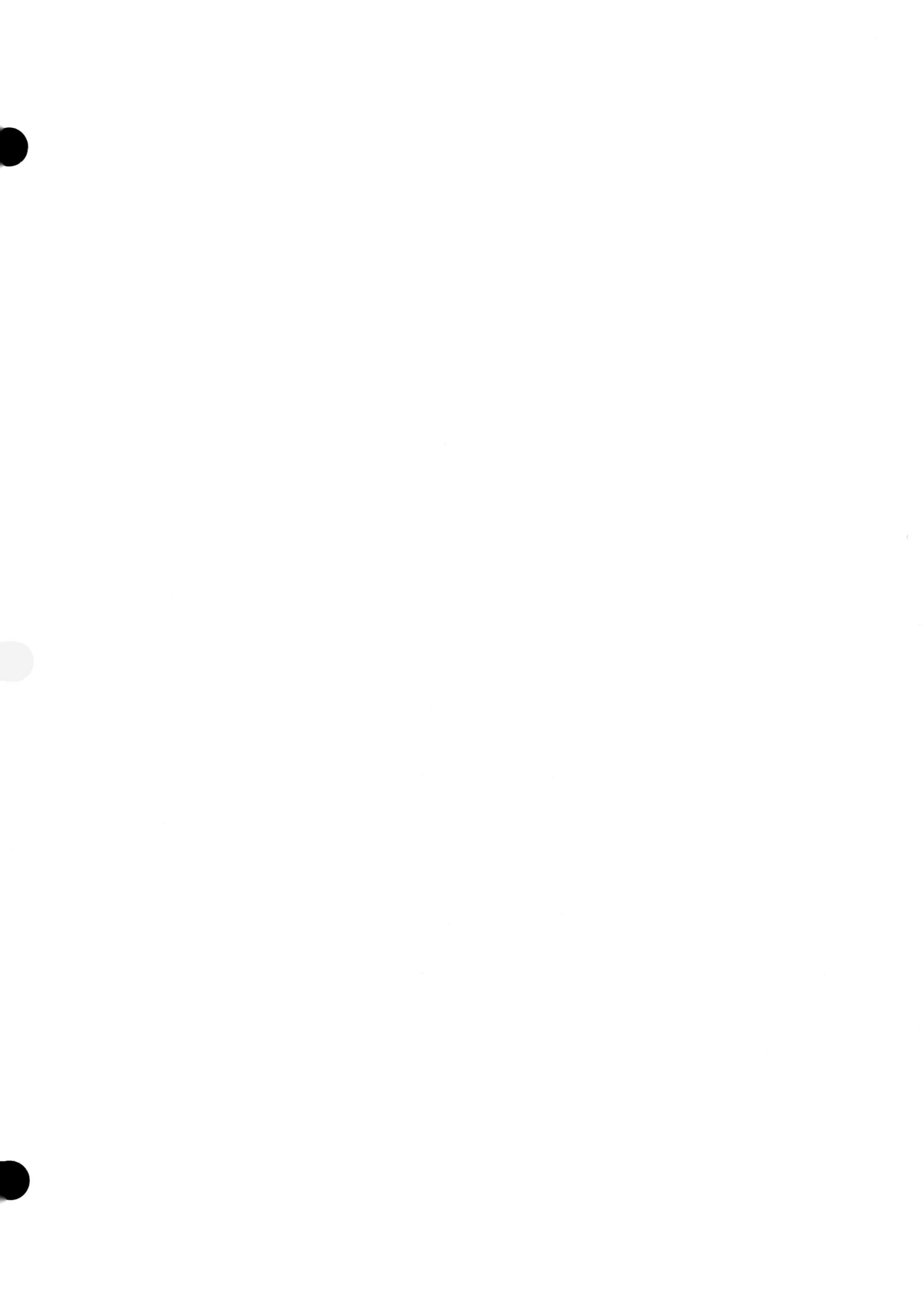

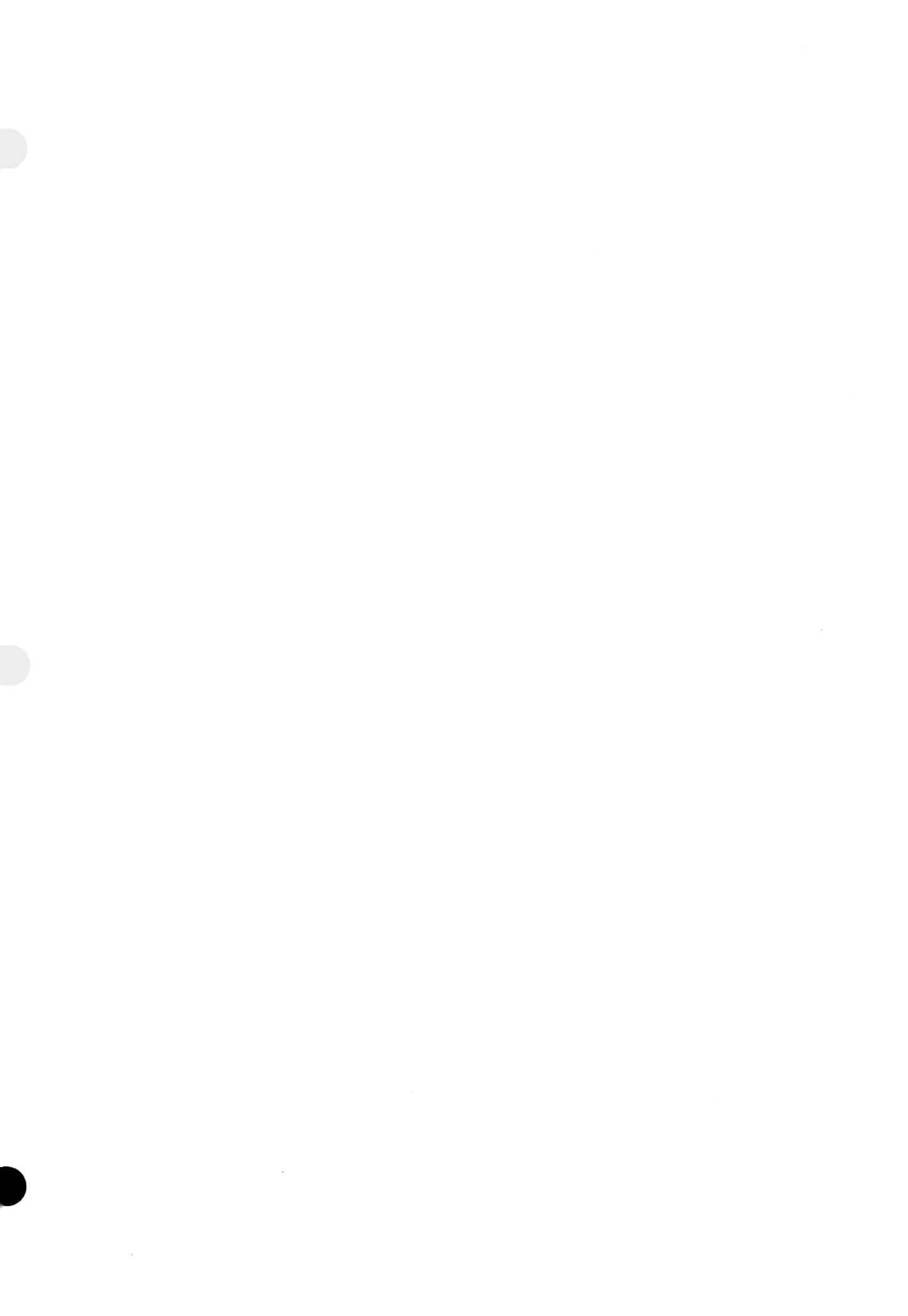

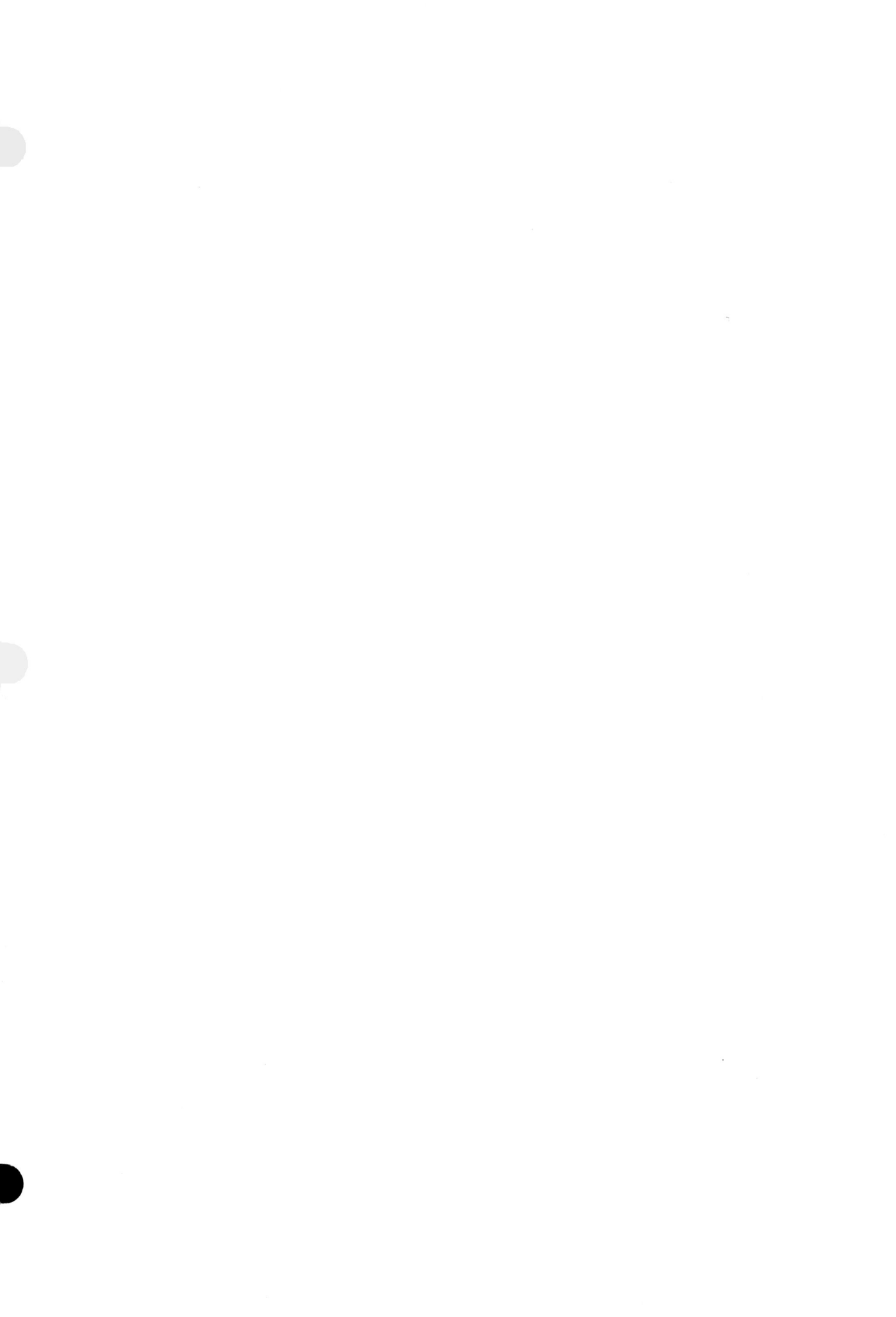